Praise for *New Hope for People with Bipolar Disorder*

"This well-documented book offers solid medical information as well as useful tips on self-awareness, maintaining relationships, and overcoming stigma. Bipolar readers, their loved ones, and health professionals will find empathy, compassion, and optimism."

> —ADA P. KAHN, PH.D., author of *Stress A–Z Sourcebook for Facing Everyday Challenges*

"This book delivers its promise. If everyone would read it, so much of the stigma that inhibits sufferers from seeking treatment would dissipate, and shame would be transformed to compassion."

> —SOL WACHTLER, former Chief Judge of New York and author of *After the Madness: A Judge's Own Prison Memoir*

"A magnificent book! This deserves the highest marks for a work on manic-depressive illness. It is profoundly engrossing, comprehensive, and its uniqueness is its message of 'hope' delivered from three distinct perspectives."

> —ARTHUR M. PETACQUE, investigative reporter, 1974 Pulitzer Prize–winner

"This creative, authoritative, state-of-the-art book is an enormously valuable tool dealing with depression and demoralization (major problems of bipolar disorder). Written from three unique perspectives, it is certain to profoundly impact the lives of patients and their families. The authors provide the latest information about bipolar disorder and depression, including the most current treatment advances with medications and psychotherapy. Above all, they present experiences of patients who have survived this illness and live productive, heroic, and inspirational lives. The bottom line: Proper diagnosis and treatment can make all the difference. No one should feel shame or let mental illness define their life!"

> —MARTIN KELLER, M.D., professor and chairman, Department of Psychiatry and Human Behavior, Brown University

Also by Jan Fawcett

Springhouse Physician's Drug Handbook, 8th Edition

Textbook of Treatment Algorithms in Psychopharmacology

Psychopharmacology and Psychotherapy: Strategies for Maximizing Treatment Outcomes, Vol. 1

Anhedonia and Affect Deficit States

The Encyclopedia of Mental Health

Also by Nancy Rosenfeld

Just As Much a Woman: Your Personal Guide to Hysterectomy and Beyond

Unfinished Journey: From Tyranny to Freedom

New Hope

FOR PEOPLE WITH

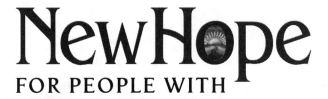

Bipolar Disorder

Jan Fawcett, M.D.,
Bernard Golden, Ph.D., and Nancy Rosenfeld

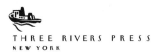

THREE RIVERS PRESS
NEW YORK

Published by Three Rivers Press, New York, New York.
Member of the Crown Publishing Group, a division of Random House, Inc.
www.randomhouse.com

THREE RIVERS PRESS and the Tugboat design are registered trademarks of Random House, Inc.

Originally published by Prima Publishing, Roseville, California, in 2001.

DISCLAIMER
This book contains general reference information about bipolar disorder in adults and children. It is not intended as a substitute for the advice of a trained clinician. Readers need to consult an appropriate medical or mental health professional before starting any medication discussed in this book. The authors and publisher are not responsible for any adverse effects resulting from information contained in this book.

Interior design by Peri Poloni, Knockout Design
Illustrations by Laurie Baker-McNeile
Author photo courtesy of Martin E. Rosenfeld

All products mentioned in this book are trademarks of their respective companies.

Printed in the United States of America

Library of Congress Cataloging-in-Publication Data
Fawcett, Jan.
    New hope for people with bipolar disorder / Jan Fawcett, Bernard Golden, Nancy Rosenfeld.
        Includes bibliographical references and index.
    1. Manic-depressive illness. 2. Depression, Mental. I. Golden, Bernard. II. Rosenfeld,
Nancy. III. Title.

RC516.F39 2000
616.89'5—dc21   00-044127

ISBN 0-7615-3008-8

10 9 8 7 6

First Edition

To Katie. Love has been described in many ways. Being able to share, appreciate, and enjoy one another's drive toward meaning is a love that the fortunate enjoy. To have a partner who can appreciate, mutually enjoy, and encourage efforts to create something worthwhile—at the same time knowing that the very activity is taking time, energy, and attention that could be available to the relationship—is a form of love that few are capable of expressing.

—JAN FAWCETT

To Dale.

—BERNARD GOLDEN

To Marty, my best friend and life partner, who once again survived another book venture. I could not have completed this task without his steadfast love and patience.

—NANCY ROSENFELD

Contents

Foreword

BIPOLAR ILLNESS HAS long been a source of fascination in the mental health field. The fascination stems from the dramatically different states of mania and depression, which are alternating yet integral components of the same illness and yet often occur simultaneously; the sudden and dramatic processes by which intense depression becomes mania literally overnight, as if a switch had been turned on; the challenge to understand how the same drug (lithium) can bring mania down and lift depression up; and finally, the paradox that in bipolar disorder, arguably the most genetic and therefore the most biological of all the mental illnesses, the psychosocial environment appears to activate the genetic vulnerability, converting it into a lifelong illness.

These features are ample reason for the growing interest among mental health professionals and brain scientists, but what of the recent surge in interest among the general public? To understand this we might turn to another fascinating character of the illness: For many bipolar patients, the dark cloud of the illness is leavened by silver linings—creativity, intelligence, and drive. As a result, the bipolar spectrum is a more frequent phenomenon among those in the public eye: artists, performers, writers, composers, and charismatic leaders.

Of course, this has long been true. So why the explosion of public interest now? The answer, I believe, is both complex and simple. Decades of research investment, principally by the National Institute of Mental Health and the pharmaceutical industry, have yielded effective treatments for many people with bipolar illness, which means there are hundreds of thousands of bipolar patients leading successful and productive lives. In so doing, each of them sends a powerful and de-stigmatizing message, especially if they are in the public eye.

Not surprisingly, popular books have been the major vehicle increasing public interest, thereby expanding the market for more books. And there has been a plethora of books. So far, what's out there falls into one of two categories: books by professionals and books by a patient or a family member.

With the appearance of this book, a new genre has been established—a close collaboration between a bipolar patient and doctors. Jan Fawcett, one of the two doctors collaborating on this book, is one of the world's leading authorities on depression and bipolar disorder. The result of this unique collaboration? First, it is a book that vibrates with the flesh and blood of real people—principally, coauthor Nancy Rosenfeld and her story, supplemented by detailed stories and quotes from well-known people with the illness. Nancy at moments seems to jump off the pages, right into your heart. At the same time, the reader is treated to a scientifically sophisticated discussion of bipolar illness—its genetics, biology, and psychology along with its psychosocial impact and pharmacological and psychotherapeutic treatments.

There is no wall between the author/patient and her two coauthors/doctors. The way her story and her reflections are woven with the scientific and professional material paints a compelling portrait of the patient as a full collaborator in advancing the understanding and treatment of her illness. This itself is an important message for the public to absorb.

The book delivers another powerful message, both explicitly and implicitly, that patients need not be defined by their illness. Every one of them is a unique person with their own personality, life experience, strengths, and weaknesses. The authors send this message by using bipolar illness as a springboard to examine various aspects of the human condition—from suggestions for managing stress, advice about sexual happiness, and optimum experience ("flow," or total involvement in life) to strategies for enhancing self-awareness and achieving job satisfaction to a nicely accessible explanation of how cognitive psychotherapy works.

While venturing into these broader areas, the book remains true to its primary focus on the key issues in bipolar disorder: its genetic and biological basis; how psychosocial stress can alter its course; the problems of substance abuse, self-stigmatization, and compliance; the impact of the illness on family, friends, and career; and, of course, state-of-the-art treatment strategies.

The authors are especially to be commended for giving particular emphasis to childhood bipolar disorder and to the issue of suicide, each of which is assigned its own chapter. Only recently has it begun to dawn on our field that the conventional wisdom that bipolar disorder rarely occurs in childhood is a myth. Likewise, for decades, the field of suicidology, spearheaded predominantly by sociologists, overlooked the fact that the great majority of suicides occur in the context of a major psychiatric disorder, principally major depression and bipolar illness. In my opinion, Jan Fawcett is our field's leading authority on suicide and the author of the most definitive study of the clinical features of depression that can predict this tragic outcome. Having this information greatly increases the chance of preventing suicide. In addition, new hope that this ultimate tragedy can be averted comes from a recent review of 28 separate reports involving more than 16,000 patients. The review concludes that the suicide rate among bipolar patients treated with lithium is six to eight times lower than it is among bipolar patients not on lithium. This is the first large-scale demonstration in psychiatry that a specific treatment can actually save lives, and it's appropriately noted in this book.

A final note. It's fair to ask how this unique collaborative effort came about and how it so clearly succeeded. I have a one-word answer: Nancy. Her boundless, almost hypomanic energy and enthusiasm were the engines, and her vision was the glue. So, Nancy's own "silver linings" made it happen. What better way to teach the public about what's possible for people with bipolar disorder who have the courage to get into treatment and stick with it, working to improve their physical and emotional health every day.

—Frederick K. Goodwin, M.D.

director of the Psychopharmacology Research Center

George Washington University Medical Center

Washington, D.C.

Acknowledgments

THIS BOOK WAS Nancy Rosenfeld's idea. The first time I met Nancy, she outlined her idea for a book about coping with bipolar disorder and asked me to write a chapter on diagnosis. I supported the idea of a book by someone who had experienced this illness, and agreed. The next thing I realized, I had written this and three more chapters.

Somehow Nancy had convinced me to become a coauthor along with Bernie Golden, whom I met and enjoyed working with in the course of producing the book. How did this happen? Nancy, the person who carries the "stigmatized" diagnosis, brought together, cajoled, and motivated two other people, with somewhat different perspectives but a common interest in reducing stigma and increasing awareness and hope with regard to bipolar disorder, to write this book.

Perhaps this is an example of the creative energy and determination that goes way beyond the concept of bipolar illness (this book wouldn't have happened without it). This is the lesson behind the message of the book. A person can become so much more than their illness. I've made two new friends and I hope our work will help people with bipolar illness and their families become informed consumers of services and see the possibilities for productive and meaningful lives.

—Jan Fawcett

* * *

Completing this book marks the end of an extremely rewarding journey and collaboration. I am extremely grateful to Nancy Rosenfeld for inviting me to participate in this project. I thank her for her vision and courage. I am appreciative of her determination, commitment to quality, and for the many moments of personal joy I experienced as part of this team. Nancy started with a story and finished with a true message of hope. My deepest appreciation goes to Dr. Patricia Robbins for her thoughtful consideration and confidence in recommending me to Nancy.

A special thanks to Jan Fawcett for his enthusiasm, knowledge, energy, and sense of calmness and centeredness that he brought to this endeavor. Frederick K. Goodwin, who spent countless hours reading and rereading our manuscript, also offered invaluable feedback, encouragement, and support.

Martha Hellander, executive director of Child and Adolescent Bipolar Foundation (CABF) provided us with parent interviews. This proved to be an invaluable source of material for chapter 11, "A Special Concern: Childhood/Adolescent Bipolar Illness."

My friends and colleagues listened to my ideas and offered critical feedback and encouragement. I also want to express my gratitude to Prima Publishing for their enthusiastic confidence in the value of this book.

Finally, my sincere appreciation to all the clients who have shared their journeys with me.

—Bernie Golden

* * *

From first conception, the writing of this book was a team effort and could not have been achieved without everyone's total commitment. I wish to thank my coauthors, Jan Fawcett and Bernie Golden, for their dedicated help, abiding loyalty, and steadfast willingness to go that extra mile. The strength of our teamwork could best be compared to a healthy and successful marriage. I recall a comment that I made to my coauthors at one meeting, "If this is work, who needs entertainment?"

A book of this nature, one that touches every aspect of the human soul, would have been impossible for me to author had it not been for the love and understanding of my husband, Marty. His patience was tested on many occasions, but each time he responded with unwavering loyalty and support.

I am deeply grateful to Frederick K. Goodwin for his substantial contribution. Besides providing the foreword, Dr. Goodwin offered indispensable critical feedback and guidance. It was his intention from the very beginning that this book meet all standards of professional excellence. His tome, *Manic-Depressive Illness* (Goodwin/Jamison), reached ultimate acclaim by the Association of American Publishers: "Most Outstanding Book, Bio- and Medical Sciences, 1990."

Deborah Bullwinkel, former program director of National Depressive and Manic-Depressive Association (National DMDA), introduced me to several key people when I first began this book venture. National DMDA became an invaluable source of research material and information throughout the writing of this book. A special thanks to the staff!

Finally, my most sincere appreciation to the staff at Prima Publishing. After working with Prima on my last book, I instinctively knew that this house, once again, would be the proper home. Jamie Miller, acquisitions editor; Alice Feinstein, editorial director; Marjorie Lery, project editor; Stephanie Marohn, copy editor; and Ben Dominitz, Prima's founder, CEO, and chairman—thank you all!

—Nancy Rosenfeld

Introduction

THIS BOOK IS THE collaborative effort of three people, each of whom approaches the subject of bipolar disorder from a distinct vantage point: Jan Fawcett, a renowned psychiatrist and psychopharmacologist; Bernard Golden, a psychologist and professor of psychology; and Nancy Rosenfeld, a woman who lives with bipolar disorder.

The uniqueness of this book is its multidimensional approach to bipolar illness rather than a concentration on a single perspective. We address the subject clinically, personally, and with an educational emphasis. Our main purpose is to bridge the gap between those of us who are afflicted and those who live around us by opening new areas of communication and, thereby, increasing each other's awareness and understanding.

Dr. Jan Fawcett, who is eminently qualified as a forerunner in the field of depression and manic-depression, details the diagnosis, biology, and treatment of bipolar disorder as well as medical strategies and risk factors for suicide. Dr. Fawcett includes the latest psychiatric findings and treatment models.

Dr. Bernard Golden focuses on the stigma of mental illness; cognitive therapy; and optimism, hope, and transcendence. In addition, Dr. Golden offers a professional analysis of Nancy's probing questions: How do we, who live with bipolar disorder, appear to others and how do we affect people who live around us? Dr. Golden also addresses the family, which is too often the forgotten link in the wellness plan. While everyone's attention is focused on the one who is ill, the rest of the family is frequently left to survive on its own.

Readers who have bipolar disorder can identify with Nancy, whose experiences are threaded throughout the book. We also cite other cases, some interesting vignettes of people whose stories illustrate points that are emphasized in each chapter.

A Message from Dr. Fawcett

Bipolar disorder can be one of the most devastating and life-threatening illnesses, yet with proper diagnosis and treatment those who have the illness can lead very creative and meaningful lives. This positive paradox is the message of this book and is exemplified by coauthor Nancy Rosenfeld, a person with the disorder.

My own contribution is a discussion of the diagnostic subtypes of the disorder, genetic aspects, the importance of a complete history, and the role of stigma—how it obscures a correct diagnosis. I cover the range of medications available, new psychiatric findings, and cutting-edge treatment models as well as common concerns and questions about the use of medication. Lastly, I address the issue of suicide, a risk in bipolar disorder, and ways in which this risk can be reduced by treatment, caring friends, and loved ones.

As authors, we combined our efforts to address the concerns, questions, and considerable range of helpful options available to the bipolar patient. This book should help inform patients, family members, and loved ones in dealing with bipolar disorder.

A Message from Dr. Golden

Both as a psychologist and as a professor, my passion resides in helping individuals expand their awareness to improve the quality of their lives. This I try to accomplish with sensitivity, respect, and clarity of communication. With these concerns in mind, we, in writing this book, practiced C.A.R.E. (Compassion, Advocacy, Recognition, and Education). Specifically:

Compassion—being sympathetic to, and helping others be sympathetic to, the pain of another.

Advocacy—individual or group activity that both empowers and is an expression of empowerment.

Recognition—those with bipolar illness must step forward to give a "face" to the illness.

Education—our primary goal, the number-one tool with which we can present facts to eliminate fear and ignorance.

We hope you experience our care!

A Message from Nancy Rosenfeld

As an author and researcher, I have devoted more than ten years to studying bipolar disorder in order to more fully understand and resolve my own issues. I have struggled with some of the same problems that you, the reader, may face. One of the biggest impediments to overcome was "stigma." Unfortunately, the public image of mental illness has been greatly influenced by a general lack of knowledge. Those of us who have suffered from mental disorders have been made to feel deviant or somewhat flawed.

I wrote this book to provide you with those answers and tools that have proven most valuable in my personal journey to wellness. Together, with my team of experts, we hope to help you achieve a smoother journey to health and well-being.

CHAPTER 1

Living with Bipolar Disorder

Is it possible to turn suffering into genuine human achievement? Nancy Rosenfeld now answers yes to this question, but it took her many years of struggling before she arrived at this answer. She was well into adulthood—married, with two grown children and a grandchild—before she came to an understanding of the positive aspects of her illness.

A question she often asked herself over the years was, Why is life unfair to people who don't deserve to suffer? In her search for an answer, she found Rabbi Harold Kushner, whose son Aaron died just two days after his fourteenth birthday from progeria, a condition that produces rapid aging. After Aaron's death, Kushner explored this question in his book *When Bad Things Happen to Good People*. The rabbi wrote, "God gave me the strength and wisdom to take my personal sorrow and forge it into an instrument of redemption which would help others." In the wake of a personal tragedy, he discovered the resiliency of the human soul. Through strength and courage, Kushner rebuilt his life. Rabbi Kushner became an inspiration to Nancy.

Nobody is promised a life free of pain and disappointment, but our capacity for strength and courage enables us to survive the tragedies and unfairness of life. Although bad things don't happen for a good reason, Rabbi Kushner found meaning in the experience of them. Human beings are complex creatures, and if life was free of pain and sorrow we would have no way to measure and test our strength and to explore the outer limits of our capabilities. We live in an imperfect world, but we, too, are imperfect. Even acceptance of our own mortality enhances the meaning of life and, as Kushner reflected, gives each of us the opportunity to be productive and to impact others so we'll be remembered as having contributed to life. Knowing that our time is limited gives value to the things we do.

Can we who are afflicted with bipolar disorder, a mental illness characterized by alternating periods of manic and depressive behavior, accept our own frailty and imperfections? Are we prepared to meet rejection from others who don't understand our dilemma? Can we assume responsibility for our disorder without using it as an excuse for our actions? Regardless of any pain dealt us in life, can we focus on the positive and forget the negative?

Many individuals who have suffered harshly have learned to survive great losses and find new ways of living full and productive lives despite their misfortune. How does one cope with a grave illness, a disabling accident, disfiguring surgery that involves loss of body parts, the death of a loved one, or shame and humiliation?

> It's possible to transform a serious loss or human tragedy, such as receiving a diagnosis of bipolar disorder, into a positive and meaningful life experience by understanding and mastering the principles of a positive mental attitude.

You will discover that it's possible to transform a serious loss or human affliction, such as receiving a diagnosis of bipolar disorder, into a positive and meaningful life experience by understanding and mastering the principles of a positive mental attitude. The human mind is resilient and capable of reversing a negative situation despite its pain and cruelty. By learning how to live again, notwithstanding seemingly insurmountable obstacles, people can emerge stronger, more self-reliant and with new goals and a new purpose in life.

Paraplegics, who have lost the use of limbs, have rediscovered their ability to lead fulfilling, productive lives. Others who have lost their sight or hearing have gained a deeper sense of perception, which does not depend on their eyes or ears, in the aftermath of their loss. Likewise, many who are afflicted with bipolar disorder have risen above the illness by adjusting to a new lifestyle.

A diagnosis of bipolar disorder, which is also known as manic-depression, can leave permanent scars. People with the disorder feel branded or stigmatized. The illness carries a bad connotation; it sounds awful and can be frightening. The mere mention of bipolar, or any mental illness, can adversely affect relationships, summoning as it does visions of the most severe forms of emotional disturbance. At the same time, each individual has a unique personality that influences his or her attitudes and conclusions regarding a given diagnosis, so everyone reacts differently.

A recent survey conducted by the National Depressive and Manic-Depressive Association (National DMDA), the organization which Jan Fawcett helped found in 1986, concluded that over 1.5 percent of the adult population in the United States (more than 2.5 million people) suffer from manic-depression.

> Nobody is immune— young or old, rich or poor. People from all walks of life are vulnerable, and bipolar disorder has confronted high-profile individuals in all fields of endeavor.

Nobody is immune—young or old, rich or poor. People from all walks of life are vulnerable, and bipolar disorder has confronted high-profile individuals in all fields of endeavor. The revelations of these people clearly indicate that financial resources, status, gender, intellect, and even the devotion of friends and family cannot prevent the illness. In their candor they reflect exceptional courage and boldness, and their disclosures are gifts.

Many celebrated individuals have educated us, helped to reduce the stigma surrounding bipolar disorder, and helped those of us who believe we are alone feel less alone. In addition, they have offered us hope that through openness and compassion we can more easily make sense of a mental illness such as manic-depression. In this book, we will meet these people and discover how they have learned to cope with their illnesses—from unipolar depression to bipolar disorder. Here, they candidly reveal their stories, specific symptoms, personal concerns, and reactions to being diagnosed with a mental illness.

JUDGE SOL WACHTLER: ON THE OTHER SIDE OF THE BENCH

One such example of a powerful personality who suffered from bipolar disorder is Judge Sol Wachtler. Judge Wachtler began his government career in 1963 when he was first elected to the city council of North Hempstead, New York. Wachtler advanced to the New York State Supreme Court in 1968 and, in 1972, was elected to the Court of Appeals, New York's highest court. In 1985, Governor Mario Cuomo appointed Wachtler chief judge of the State of New York and the Court of Appeals. In an editorial piece for the *New York Times*, Alan Dershowitz wrote, "Sol Wachtler was not a good judge . . . he was a great judge."

Just as Judge Wachtler was on the threshold of becoming governor of New York, a cherished dream, he became instead Sol Wachtler, federal prisoner, assigned to solitary confinement. How did this happen?

The story of Sol Wachtler is one of illicit love and clandestine meetings, compulsive behavior and drug abuse, rejection and deceit, shame and self-reproach, depression with an attempt to self-medicate, and the fear of stigma—of being branded mentally incompetent.

Although it was a reckless act of compulsive behavior that abruptly led to Wachtler's self-destruction and ultimate fall, the root of Sol Wachtler's problem was his bipolar illness. It wasn't until 1992 that Judge Wachtler finally received the diagnosis of bipolar disorder, but by then his unchecked illness had destroyed his professional career and his life.

Though he made a courageous comeback from the abyss into which he had plunged, he dismisses any sentiments regarding the achievement. "I don't feel as if I've reclaimed my life," Wachtler says. "I've got a long way to go, and it will never be the same as before. I will always have deep scars. Take, for example, the times I hear myself talking to my students about 'my' court. But suddenly I realize that it no longer *is* my court. It *was* my court for 25 years, but that's all gone now."

Five years after his diagnosis with bipolar disorder, Judge Wachtler went public in a book about his experiences, *After the Madness: A Judge's Own Prison Memoir*. He maintained his dignity and sense of humor without excusing the actions that resulted in his arrest and conviction. Judge Wachtler's personal story can serve as a deterrent to others, as well as an inspiration.

> Just as Judge Wachtler was on the threshold of becoming governor of New York, a cherished dream, he became instead Sol Wachtler, federal prisoner.

There is no debating the pathological nature of manic-depressive illness. The disorder can unquestionably destroy lives, not to mention relationships. At the same time, the energy and the creativity that spills forth from this otherwise devastating condition can yield dividends for the afflicted and those who witness their lives.

Judge Wachtler flew to Chicago for a personal interview with Nancy, Bernie Golden, and Deborah Bullwinkel.[1] At that time, Wachtler was teaching law again, twice a week, at a small college in New York while working at a mediation firm, writing his next book, and traveling extensively to lecture about bipolar disorder and his experience. Here is Sol Wachtler's personal account of his fall from grace.

Judge Wachtler was incarcerated in September 1993 for harassing his former mistress. At that time, he was a walking time bomb and was placed in solitary confinement for two weeks under close observation. The second and only other time that Wachtler was confined to solitary was for his own protection, after he was stabbed by another prison inmate. Although Wachtler never condoned his deviant behavior, it is clear that his bipolar disorder and abuse of prescription drugs contributed to his wrongdoing.

"Don't misunderstand," said Wachtler. "Bipolar is not, and should not be, an excuse for criminal conduct. If someone afflicted with the disorder commits a criminal act, that person should be stopped or arrested before more harm is done."

Wachtler's eminent position in the outer world did not earn him special treatment in jail. He was subjected to all the forms of inhumanity prisoners endure, including strip searches. During imprisonment, what he longed for most was privacy and freedom. "This loss was far greater than power or prestige," he said.

"Prison was tough. Everything and every day was a constant reminder that I was a prisoner behind bars—the guards, the keys, mail call. At one time I considered suicide, but quickly ruled it out as a viable alternative. Suicide takes courage, but I had none."

"It took more courage to live," observed Nancy.

"Perhaps. But I was stuck in the here and now, and with no future image. I saw nothing beyond life in prison. Days were endless, and each seemed like eternity. All thoughts were negative. I worried about what I'd do when I got out and how I'd make a living. I was also a patient in the mental health unit, and the treatment there was deplorable." Wachtler credits Prozac with keeping him going during his 13-month incarceration.

After his release, Wachtler had to contend with the views of others about what he had done. "Subtle things happened which were hurtful," he said. "For example, as former chief judge of New York I was invited to attend the presentation of an award to Ruth Ginsburg, a justice of the United States Supreme Court. Before the actual ceremony, recognition was extended to all distinguished former recipients of that award who were in attendance. I listened and waited, but my name was never called. I checked the program, then discovered that it had been omitted from the list."

"As if you never existed," said Deborah.

"Yes. Like a blot in history that was simply erased," he replied. "Around the same time, Mike Wallace invited me to do a segment of *60 Minutes*, but I declined."

"Why?" asked Nancy.

"He can be very rough," said Wachtler.

"What about your relationship today with Governor Cuomo?" said Nancy. "I know the two of you had been friends for years, but the friendship disintegrated and you sued him."

In 1991, Judge Sol Wachtler had filed a summons and complaint against Governor Cuomo in *Wachtler v. Cuomo*. The governor had threatened to cut the newly proposed budget of the state court system, which Wachtler had submitted to the legislature. At that time, Wachtler felt he "could not permit" Cuomo's budget cuts because of the damaging effect he believed they would have on the court system.

"There's been a warming since then," said Wachtler, with a smile. "Just two weeks ago we lunched together, and Mario confided, 'Once you sued me, I knew you were crazy.'"

"How did you view your illness?" inquired Bernie.

"Bizarre," said Wachtler. "But at that time I didn't consider my behavior strange. I thought *they* [others] were bizarre, not me. 'I'm not talking too fast,' I'd say. 'You're listening too slowly.' Looking back, I don't see how I could have entertained that thought pattern. It's incomprehensible."

In his memoir, Wachtler sums up manic behavior, and the unrealistic overconfidence and grandiosity that accompany full-blown mania: "Have a speech to deliver? I don't have to prepare—my head is full of the world's greatest speeches—just give me a platform."[2]

> At the time I didn't consider my behavior strange. I thought they [others] were bizarre, not me. "I'm not talking too fast," I'd say. "You're listening too slowly."
>
> —JUDGE SOL WACHTLER

On the other end of the spectrum, he describes his state of mind at the height of depression as like the inner surface of an abyss. The physical manifestations of his depression included loss of appetite, constant weeping, sleeplessness, and fluttering in his stomach.

Before his diagnosis, he had convinced himself that he was suffering from a brain tumor. An MRI (magnetic resonance imaging) scan in 1992, however, revealed no brain tumor, but showed UBOs (unidentified bright objects) in the right parietal region of his brain. The significance of UBOs, as Kay Jamison reveals in her book, *An Unquiet Mind*, is the scientific conclusion that bipolar disorder is a biological condition involving changes in brain chemistry (see chapter 3).

> It's important for anyone with mental illness to recognize the need for professional guidance before behavior turns antisocial. Not to seek help is foolish.
>
> —JUDGE SOL WACHTLER

"It's important for anyone with mental illness to recognize the need for professional guidance before behavior turns antisocial," cautioned Wachtler. "Not to seek help is foolish, stupid, terribly destructive. My wife, a trained certified social worker, pleaded with me to get counseling." Wachtler eventually did, and Prozac freed him. "Had I accepted my wife's advice earlier, today I'd be governor of New York."

Wachtler resisted psychiatric help because of the stigma society imposes on those who "seek to remedy a defect of the mind." He recalled the lesson of Thomas Eagleton, the former United States senator and 1972 vice-presidential candidate who was dropped from the ballot after the information was leaked that he had once received psychiatric treatment.

Psychotherapy helped Wachtler, and he still sees his psychiatrist regularly. "I'm on a maintenance program, but I also self-assess. I measure what I've done and how I've done it. For example, am I speaking too rapidly? I keep a reality checklist." As for physical exercise, which also helps regulate mood, Wachtler takes long walks.

Looking back on the behavior that resulted in his public disgrace, Wachtler sees how out of control he was.

"I didn't realize the absurdity of my actions toward her [his mistress] until after I started on Prozac. I had low-level depression and mania prior to the relationship, but I was unaware of how ridiculous it was until later. Then I was helped to make sense of why I had sought out the relationship in the first place. I remember my wife's comment once that if ever I had an affair, she didn't want to know about it. But then she read about my affair on page one of the *New York Times*."

"Do you worry about depression returning?" asked Bernie.

"Constantly. As soon as I see it happening, I return to the doctor so he can adjust my medication."

At the end of the interview, Nancy commented that everything happens for a reason. "No!" Wachtler exclaimed, then added, "You have no idea how many people have told me that. But I can't accept it."

Bernie and Nancy were left to speculate on the reasons for the vehemence of Wachtler's last remark. The judge was approaching his seventieth birthday, and his very identity had been based on his judicial career and becoming the governor of New York. Now all that was gone; his dreams had turned to ashes. Not for several months would Wachtler reveal the reasons behind his vehement reaction that day in Chicago.

Since Wachtler's release from prison six years ago he has waged a crusade to help other people who, like himself, are afflicted with mental disorders. He travels extensively across the country lecturing about his bipolar condition. "Get help," he advocates. "Don't be stupid like I was." But, by reaching out to others in the hope of removing the stigma of mental illness he has positioned himself for public attack.

During a recent address in Albany, New York, Wachtler informed his audience that more people with mental illnesses are in prison today than are in hospitals receiving treatment. "Nobody is cured in prison," he said. "They become more dysfunctional." But, the very next day his words made headline news: *New York: "Ex-con Talks About Prison Experience."*

"Why talk," said Wachtler, "if every time it's like putting a pencil in my own eye. I'm not proud of having been in prison. But, to refer to me as an 'ex-con' rather than by name or as the former chief judge is a constant bad reminder, like waking up a sleeping dog."

Wachtler still maintains a busy schedule with all his pursuits and, as a mental health advocate, educating others is at the forefront of his concern. Nevertheless, Sol Wachtler has permanently lost "his court."

MIKE WALLACE: LIVING WITH THE BLACK DOG

Mike Wallace, veteran news correspondent of *60 Minutes* since the show first aired in 1968, is another well-known personality who suffered from a mental disorder. In his case, it was depression, which Winston Churchill, a fellow sufferer, referred to as "the black dog." Churchill's black dog image of a depressive episode profoundly illustrates the all-consuming desolation experienced by people in this mental state.

Journalism's legendary tough guy, Wallace was shadowed with his first bout of depression after General William Westmoreland named him in a $120 million libel suit against CBS. "The Uncounted Enemy: A Vietnam Deception," a 1982 *CBS News Reports* documentary anchored by Wallace, charged Westmoreland with "cooking the books" in Vietnam in 1967 by failing to inform the American people of the truth regarding the number of enemy troops still fighting and how many more were coming down from North Vietnam to help drive the Americans out of the country.[3]

Fear of the stigma surrounding depression made Mike Wallace afraid of losing his job as CBS news correspondent and anchorman. He felt it necessary, at all costs, to maintain his macho image.

In 1984, two years after Wallace's CBS documentary aired, when he accused Westmoreland of falsifying reports to the American public, Wallace began an 18-week trial. It was a tough time for him as he was forced to sit helplessly by while being branded a "cheat" and a "liar." He was also trying to do his job, working nights and going off for a couple days at a time on a shoot. Because of his inability to concentrate on anything else, he endured sleepless nights, weight loss, and depression so severe that he described himself as "feeling lower than a snake's belly."[4] Throughout this period, Wallace felt so ashamed at the prospect of being branded with the stigma of mental illness that he attempted to mask his feelings from everyone. Fear of the stigma surrounding depression made him afraid of losing his job as a CBS news correspondent and anchorman. He felt it necessary, at all costs, to maintain his macho image.

While shame and guilt are typically components of depression, Mike Wallace's bout with depression was compounded by his tough-guy image. It was the meaning he gave to the illness (that depression is like a black hole), combined with his severe and unrealistically high self-expectations, that further exacerbated his shame and depression.

When Wallace was first diagnosed, he did not consider the public's reaction. He was too sick to care, and yet he didn't want to lose his job. He believed people knew something strange was going on, but they didn't know what it was. At that time, neither did Wallace. Not until later did he become aware of public opinion. When out in public places, he imagined that everyone was pointing at him, saying, "There's the cheat, the fraud, the fake."[5]

By the time Mike Wallace was hospitalized and diagnosed with clinical depression, he was grateful to have some kind of diagnosis. He had worried that he had a brain tumor or that he was losing his mind.

Wallace couldn't sleep, and because of his insomnia he started taking half a sleeping pill. From half it went up to one sleeping pill, and then if he still wasn't sleeping, he'd take another. He felt miserable all day long.

Wallace recalls his anguished calls to his personal physician. "I was really talking suicide and he would say, 'C'mon, Mike, you're not going to do that. You're strong and capable. This, too, shall pass.'"[6]

By the time Wallace was hospitalized and diagnosed with clinical depression, he was grateful to have some kind of diagnosis. Like Sol Wachtler, he had worried that he had a brain tumor or, alternatively, that he was losing his mind. But the pain associated with Wallace's clinical depression was more painful than Sol Wachtler's untreated manic episodes. People rarely seek help during manic episodes because they feel good. It's those who live around them, both family and friends, who suffer the most as their lives are directly affected by the manic attacks of loved ones.

Wallace was released from the hospital after one week, and sent home with a prescription for antidepressants and plenty to read on depression. Still, he remained quiet about his illness until a friend, novelist William Styron, came out of the closet about his mental health problems. Only then could Mike speak candidly about his own affliction.

> I think it's useful to talk about depression because it remains a mystery to so many people, and also verboten to so many people to talk about. If somebody has suffered it, survived it, and gone on about his business, and people know that, then it's got to be useful.
>
> —MIKE WALLACE

"I think it's useful to talk about depression because it remains a mystery to so many people, and also verboten to so many people to talk about. If somebody has suffered it, survived it, and gone on about his business, and people know that, then it's got to be useful."[7]

In 1998 HBO broadcasted a special one-hour documentary, "Dead Blue: Surviving Depression." The program featured Mike Wallace along with the Pulitzer Prize–winning author of *Sophie's Choice*, William Styron, and clinical psychologist and author of *Undercurrents*, Martha Manning. The three featured guests spoke candidly about their illness with no reportage, script, narration, or "experts." Wallace noted how depression, despite epidemic proportions, was "shrouded in secrecy—something to hide, a skeleton in the closet associated with guilt, fear, and shame." Their message: "There is a way out of the darkness."

Wallace recovered from this bout of depression, but suffered two relapses, in 1985 and 1993, before his health was fully restored. Depression-free ever since, Mike follows a strict maintenance program and returns to his doctor for semiannual checkups, which he's dubbed "lube jobs." Of his experience, he said, "I think I'm a wiser and kinder man for having been through it. That doesn't mean that I've lost the edge; I'm more empathic, more careful about making snap judgments, and I think I like myself better."[8]

COPING WITH DEPRESSION

As the daughter of famed news broadcaster Walter Cronkite, anchorman of the *CBS Evening News* (1962–1981), Kathy Cronkite has lived in the public eye all her life. Today she is a popular writer, journalist, public speaker, and one of the millions who suffer from clinical depression.

In the spring of 1990, Kathy Cronkite read an interview with Mike Wallace in *U.S. News & World Report*, in which Wallace openly talked about his battle with depression. His admission gave Cronkite the courage to face her own struggle.

"I've known Mike Wallace and his family all my life. Even when I was young, he was one of those rare grownups who seemed to take me seriously. Still, I never dreamed that as an adult I would interview him, as one professional to another."[9]

Cronkite had shared the same fear as Mike Wallace about publicly disclosing her personal battle with depression. She, too, had been worried about repercussions that any disclosure of her illness might have on her professional life. But it was the black dog that Cronkite most dreaded. "[Churchill's] black dog has really got me," she wrote in her book, *On the Edge of Darkness*. "[His] image of despair suits me better than 'the black hole.' A black hole just swallows you up. But, this dog . . . I can't cope while he's there."

Kathy Cronkite eventually admitted to being in grave danger from her depression, but not until after she had contemplated swallowing a can of liquid Drano.

Academy Award–winning actor Rod Steiger has also had suicidal tendencies. "You have moments when you're locked in an ever-increasing terror," he told Cronkite when she interviewed him for her book. "You begin to doubt your sanity. When you're depressed, there's no calendar. There are no dates, there's no day, there's no night, there's no seconds, there's no minutes, there's nothing. You're just existing in this cold, murky, ever-heavy atmosphere, like they put you inside a vial of mercury." Steiger insists that you can't understand these feelings unless you've experienced them. Yet, no matter how sick he was, Steiger felt that acting was something he could always do. "Now I realize I didn't have as much control as I thought I had." When depressed, he was "acting in a fog."[10]

> When you're de-pressed, there's no calendar. There are no dates, there's no day, there's no night, there's no seconds, there's no minutes, there's nothing.
>
> —ROD STEIGER

Unlike the others, however, Rod Steiger has not been ashamed to go public with his illness. "It might have damaged me to some degree in the profession, but across the country one in five has a mental disease. It's about time we begin to talk about this thing."[11]

Steiger believes that narcissism makes a person more vulnerable to depression. "If you've got a huge powerful ego and then all of a sudden it's proven that you're nobody but another human being, you can slide down a long way because you're way up there. I felt that I was gonna live forever. Why? Because my name's Rod Steiger."[12]

Writer Kay Redfield Jamison, who has bipolar disorder and knows the horror of deep depression intimately, describes "the black dog" in *An Unquiet Mind*:

> *Depression is awful beyond words or sounds or images. . . . It bleeds relationships through suspicion, lack of confidence and self-respect, the inability to enjoy life, to walk or talk or think normally, the exhaustion, the night terrors, the day terrors. . . . [Depression] gives you the experience of how it must be to be old, to be old and sick, to be dying; to be slow of mind; to be lacking in grace, polish, and coordination; to be ugly; to have no belief in the possibilities of life, the*

*pleasures of sex, the exquisiteness of music, or the ability to make
yourself and others laugh.*

    *Depression is flat, hollow, and unendurable . . . tiresome. People
cannot abide being around you. . . . You are tedious . . .
irritable and paranoid and humorless and lifeless and critical and
demanding and no reassurance is ever enough. You're frightened,
and you're frightening.*[13]

Like Kay Jamison, Nancy can identify with devastating episodes
of deep and disabling depression. There is no minimizing its shatter-
ing, destabilizing effects, not only on the patient, but also on family
and friends. Depression is dark days and endless nights. Trivial, mun-
dane tasks become insurmountable. Listening to music, taking a walk,
or partaking in some otherwise pleasant outing or gathering with
family or friends—none of these former pastimes bring joy to the afflicted, only sadness. All are sharp reminders of the past, a time when
life felt good. Depression has a domino effect—one defeat leads to
another and another and another. . . .

"One of the mysteries of depression," said Kathy Cronkite, "is
why people succumb when they do, why a blow that cripples one person is taken in stride by another, and why a person who has survived
great adversity is laid low by one of life's predictable stumbling
blocks." For example, Cronkite was deeply traumatized by the sudden
death of her beloved dog who was killed by a car. She had never experienced the death of a close relative or friend, and the loss of her dog
plunged her into one of the deepest and long-lasting depressive
episodes that she had ever encountered.

While it may not be apparent in everyone with manic-depression,
frequently there are psychosocial stressors, as in Cronkite's situation,
that trigger the illness in those who have a genetic predisposition
for it. Similarly, a casual observer may underestimate the severity of
emotional distress caused by such events. Fortunately, Cronkite had
the support and understanding of family and friends who were deeply

> *When the black dog of depression rides along, you're in for a roller-coaster ride of exhilaration and despair. Those of us whose marriages survive seem to agree that it is largely because we are married to extraordinary people— "angels" or "saints."*
>
> —KATHY CRONKITE

attached to their own pets and could empathize with her loss.

Cronkite is candid about her personal relationships and the destructive nature of depression. After suffering a major crisis, she feared that her marriage was in jeopardy even though her husband had stood by her throughout her ups and downs. "No marriage runs on a smooth road all the time," she said, "but when the black dog of depression rides along, you're in for a roller-coaster ride of exhilaration and despair. Those of us whose marriages survive seem to agree that it is largely because we are married to extraordinary people—'angels' or 'saints.'"[14]

NANCY'S STORY: A DESPERATE CRY FOR HELP

"I felt like an oddball growing up," said Nancy. "I didn't fit. I was Jewish in a Gentile community, tall for my age, and older than most other students in my class. Being both older and taller created a sharp contrast between 'me' and 'them,' which made me feel isolated. My basic shyness and feeling of insecurity led to hero worshiping—the popular high school cheerleader, an older cousin, a beautiful aunt. By creating a protective shield for myself I found safety in the shadow of others."

Nancy's moods continued to haunt her from childhood on. From an emotional child who had been heavily doted on as her parents' firstborn, she continued to struggle with chronic low self-esteem and depression throughout her childhood. Although her moods became less severe and less frequent as she matured, they persisted well into adulthood.

Nancy's adult life was typical of the upper-middle-class suburban American housewife of the late 1960s to early 1980s. She sublimated her individuality to raise a family while living in the shadow of her husband's career. Although she had moments of uncertainty and sadness, not until her children entered adolescence and needed her less did she begin to experience a gripping, gnawing, and growing feeling of emptiness. What finally hit home was that there must be more to life, she thought. At the same time, Nancy realized that she needed to develop her own identity. It was then, when Nancy entered her 40s, that she found her own identity as a political activist. During this period she exhibited the first signs of bipolar disorder when she became obsessively involved in the rescue of a former Soviet scientist and political prisoner.

BIPOLAR DISORDER AND CREATIVITY

Since perfection does not exist among humans, all human beings live with some kind of impairment or disability. It's how we adjust to our imperfections by learning how to cope and perhaps alter our path that determines our potential for happiness in life. When faced with challenge, what are the options?

"Is there life after manic-depression?" questioned Patty Duke, who suffers from the illness.

In looking for an answer, Duke learned that people who share her disorder are frequently highly creative and successful individuals. The very nature of bipolar disorder is conducive to high energy and imaginative thinking.

Kay Jamison, Ph.D., and Frederick K. Goodwin, M.D., have presented a reasonable theory that supports the concept of bipolar "advantages," more commonly referred to as "fluency of thinking." They have shown a high correlation between creative personalities and bipolar illness. Jamison determined that highly creative people are usually most productive and prolific during periods of hypomania. In fact, it is the very intensity of such moods that propels and inspires

Nancy: Hypomania

In the spring of 1996, at the age of 54, Nancy was admitted to the hospital for hysterectomy after being diagnosed with a uterine tumor. Her state of imbalance was immediately evident when she exhibited obvious signs of hypomanic behavior, or low-grade mania.

"The doctors and nurses kept shaking their heads, and one doctor suggested I be given lithium to control the mania," said Nancy. "But, since I realized that my manic state was only a temporary condition, I declined the doctor's 'offer.' I enjoyed the intensity of the moment, that feeling of being overly zealous." Although Nancy's laughter in the hospital was considered extreme, it probably prevented a bout with the blues. Furthermore, medicinal humor is psychologically beneficial and contributes to the healing process.

Nancy's normal daily antidepressant dosage, 50 milligrams of Zoloft, had apparently been insufficient in controlling the sudden hormonal shock to her system after a hysterectomy. Though aware of her manic state, Nancy had not been able to control it. In fact, she actually enjoyed the temporary mania.

Episode #1: Two friends, a husband and wife, stopped by to see Nancy in her hospital room, but the visit turned sour because Nancy was manicky and nearly out of control. When the husband asked Nancy what had happened during surgery to cause some "complication," she told them of the doctor's surprising discovery of an advanced case of endometriosis. The couple's reaction was anger. Apparently they had been very worried that something had gone seriously wrong because Nancy had exaggerated her condition during an earlier telephone conversation with them. Nevertheless, their emphatic response triggered an explosive reaction from Nancy.

"My alter ego began to speak," recalled Nancy. *Why on earth had this couple come to visit me if they were unable to be supportive?*

Were they disappointed I wasn't dying? Weren't visitors supposed to help buoy a patient's spirits? Should it be the patient's responsibility to guard her every word—and entertain? Isn't this nonsense?

"At the time I was furious," admitted Nancy. "I had just had surgery that morning, it had gone well, but I was lying there uncomfortably while my two friends seemed to be arguing over semantics. Now I realize that the problem stemmed from me, not them.

Episode #2: A second event occurred moments after the first. Still in pain from the first hospital encounter and her overreaction, Nancy was quickly transformed by a surge of mania. When another group of friends appeared in the doorway with cheerful faces, that was enough to cause a sudden change of mood from anger to giddiness.

"I was so happy to see my friends," said Nancy. "It was especially meaningful because they needed to travel some distance to see me in the hospital. I asked when they had made the decision to visit that evening. Dorothy replied that she had actually tried three times that day to ask me about visiting hours, but that it was hard to keep me on a single topic. I remember laughing apologetically and responding that visiting hours were all day and all night. As to the 'uplifting' experience of visiting me in the hospital after such a long trek, their response: "It's more than we bargained for, even better than 'Saturday Night Live!'"

What Nancy's friends had witnessed was a hypomanic episode. People who become hypomanic can be very entertaining and fun to be with. They laugh a lot and are very talkative and animated. They are also prone to angry outbursts and downright meanness, however, and their energy levels can climb so high that sleep and concentration become a problem.

creative thinkers. Jamison herself is an example of a highly creative and successful career person who lives with manic-depression. She did not receive a diagnosis of bipolar disorder until after she had begun her career as a psychologist. Elements of creative thinking, many of which are associated with cognitive changes that take place during mild manias as well, include:

- word fluency
- associational fluency
- expressional fluency
- ideational fluency [15]

An artistic temperament and imagination, the by-product of such creative assets, have given rise to many celebrated and distinguished individuals. Among these talented people who have bipolar disorder, we find poets, writers, artists, business tycoons, political leaders, and scientists.

Kay Jamison writes about her own experience with the illness. "I honestly believe that as a result of it I have felt more things, more deeply; had more experiences, more intensely; loved more, and been more loved; laughed more often for having cried more often; appreciated more . . . seen the finest and the most terrible in people, and slowly learned the values of caring, loyalty, and seeing things through. . . . But, normal or manic, I have run faster, thought faster, and loved faster than most I know. . . . It has made me test the limits of my mind.

> Highly creative people are usually most productive and prolific during periods of hypomania. In fact, it is the very intensity of such moods that propels and inspires creative thinkers.

"Extremes of emotions are a gift—the capacity to be passionately involved in life, to care deeply about things, to feel hurt; a lot of people don't have that. It's the transition in and out of the highs and lows, the constant contrast, that fosters creativity."[16]

Impairment, the inability to function normally, does not occur until after the hypomanic stage has progressed into full-blown mania.

Without trying to romanticize or falsely exaggerate the positives, history has proven that people afflicted with bipolar disorder are in good company. The ability to inspire is as important to public officials and world leaders as creativity is to people in the arts. Many of our most powerful men and women are among the afflicted. But not everyone who is creative or productive is manic-depressive, nor is everyone with manic-depressive illness creative.

Goodwin and Jamison list certain bipolar characteristics common to many political dignitaries, " . . . high energy, enthusiasm, intensity of emotion, persuasion by mood, charisma, contagion of spirit, gregarious and extrovertish, increased belief in one's self and one's ideas, heightened alertness and observational abilities, and risk-takers."[17]

Among the political leaders with bipolar disorder are Napoleon, Mussolini, Alexander the Great, Lord Nelson, and Oliver Cromwell, to name just a few.

Alexander Hamilton (1755–1804), first U.S. Secretary of the Treasury, suffered from extreme paranoia, hypersexuality, financial speculation and consequent indebtedness, rapid and fiery temper, extreme mood swings, and inordinate energy.

Abraham Lincoln (1809–1865) struggled with suicidal depressions; Robert E. Lee (1807–1870), intermittent depressions; Winston Churchill (1874–1965), severe periods of depression alternating with periods of high energy; and, Martin Luther (1483–1546), periods of deep psychosis and, occasionally, suicidal melancholy.[18]

According to *Time* magazine, even current success heroes of our culture such as Ted Turner (*Time*'s "Man of the Year" in 1991) reputedly use mood-stabilizing drugs.

> Extremes of emotions are a gift—the capacity to be passionately involved in life, to care deeply about things, to feel hurt; a lot of people don't have that. It's the transition in and out of the highs and lows, the constant contrast, that fosters creativity.
>
> —KAY JAMISON

Words from the Wise

The following are quotations from some famous, highly creative individuals who suffered from bipolar disorder.

"Why is it that all men who are outstanding in philosophy, poetry, or the arts are melancholic?"

—ARISTOTLE

"By our own spirits we are defied;
We poets in our youth begin in gladness;
But thereof comes in the end despondency and madness."

—WILLIAM WADSWORTH

"One must harbor chaos within oneself to give birth to a dancing star."

—NIETZSCHE

"Life is a train of moods."

—RALPH WALDO EMERSON

TIPPER GORE: DISPELLING MYTHS

"Coming out" about her illness was not easy for Tipper Gore. Yet she felt the only way of reducing the stigma of mental disorders was to educate the American public. Gore has remained silent about the details of her own illness, citing just a few examples. Her struggle with clinical depression manifested itself soon after a car accident that had nearly killed her son.[19]

It is normal for people to experience grief when something terrible happens to a loved one, or to oneself. Normal grief over a death, serious injury, or diagnosis of some catastrophic illness crosses the line and becomes "abnormal" only after it becomes apparent that one's grief has turned into prolonged sorrow, with no end in sight.

As the daughter of a woman who was twice hospitalized for depression, Tipper Gore was warned against revealing this "delicate" information to a reporter from the *New York Times*. "I think you want to dispute the fact that you had a difficult childhood," she was cautioned. "Right," said Mrs. Gore, "I had a great childhood."[20]

How does Gore maintain an even keel? What works for her is regular exercise and living with humor. "I think it's important to have a strategy for dealing with stress," she said. "I run, I roller-blade, and I bike ride. It's important for me to be outdoors as much as possible." She also cites the role of humor: "I think humor is a stress reliever, as is doing things we enjoy."[21]

Gore hoped her own story would help to dispel old myths by eliminating the need to whisper about mental illness. Her aim: to

For Art's Sake

John Berryman, the Pulitzer Prize–winning poet, described the possible benefits to his art of being a manic-depressive:

I do feel strongly that among the greatest pieces of luck for high achievement is ordeal . . . Beethoven's deafness, Goya's deafness, Milton's blindness. . . . And, I think that what happens in my poetic work will probably largely depend not on my sitting calmly on my ass. . . . But being knocked in the face, and thrown flat, and given cancer, and all kinds of other things short of senile dementia. At that point, I'm out, but short of that, I don't know. I hope to be nearly crucified.

As the daughter of a woman who was twice hospitalized for depression, Tipper Gore was warned against revealing this "delicate" information to a reporter from the New York Times. "I think you want to dispute the fact that you had a difficult childhood," she was cautioned. "Right," said Mrs. Gore, "I had a great childhood."

convince the nation that mental illness is not the result of bad parenting or lax churchgoing, but that its root is a chemical imbalance. Her problem was with her brain's "gas gauge."[22]

ROBERT BOORSTIN: HOPE FOR FUTURE ADVANCES

A colorful political figure, Robert Boorstin has struggled with bipolar disorder since his student days in college. Bernie Golden and Nancy interviewed Bob at the 1999 National DMDA Conference in Houston, Texas.

Bob was born into a well-to-do family from Beverly Hills, California. His privileged lifestyle— inherited wealth and an emphasis on high academic achievement (both father and grandfather were Yale graduates, while his mother was a Wellesley graduate who also studied at the Sorbonne)—did not replace what Bob missed most: love, peace, and family stability.

One month shy of Bob's tenth birthday, his 40-year-old father died suddenly from a massive heart attack. At the time of his father's death, Bob's parents were vacationing overseas. As he and his father had never developed a close relationship Bob was virtually unmoved by his father's death.

"My father was a driven, ambitious, and miserably unhappy man," he said. Later, Bob tried unsuccessfully to find some "emotional link" when, as an adult, he traveled to Greece to retrace his father's boyhood footsteps.

Boorstin's political career began in 1993 as a foreign policy speech writer for President Clinton. Afterwards, Bob was appointed senior adviser to the Secretary of the Treasury before resigning for private life. He still operates out of Washington and is politically active there, representing a firm that does international poll surveys. He admitted that driving up to work each morning at the White House had been very exciting, as was accompanying the president on Air Force One for his worldwide travels. Nevertheless, Bob was glad to leave the federal government behind after six-and-a-half years. It meant that he could finally speak openly about his illness.

"There was no hint of emotional illness before I was 17 or 18," he said. "Unlike my twin brother who followed the family patriarchs to Yale, I spent four enjoyable years at Harvard University studying international relations and acting as chief editor of the *Crimson* [Harvard's school newspaper]. But, I had no idea what that constant feverish pace was doing to me [emotionally]. I was very manicky at Harvard.

"Then, I went to England and did my postgraduate work at James College in Cambridge. During my first year at Cambridge, everything seemed fine. I was also dating a woman whom I liked very much. The next year I broke off my relationship with her, and afterwards I was very lonely. Besides, I hated the English atmosphere—it was cold, bleak, and it rained all the time. I cried and couldn't get out of bed. At that time, I was teaching, studying Chinese and Russian, and trying to write my dissertation. I was overloaded.

"A combustible series of events that occurred within four months' time led to the ultimate upheaval in my life. First, my stepfather's death, then the broken relationship with a woman, and finally my decision to change professions.

"My stepfather and I were very close and I loved him desperately," said Bob. "He was a very supportive and caring person." After struggling with emotional problems for several years, Bob's condition was finally diagnosed as bipolar disorder at age 24. His stepfather arrived in Cambridge to pay him a visit. "I talked, and he listened. Listening is very powerful, you know.

"I had suicidal flashes. I pictured myself dead, and that everyone would be happier without me. I also dreamed of being 'accidentally killed.' Finally, at the urging of my parents, I underwent psychoanalysis. I visited the shrink four to five days each week for two years and was never diagnosed. I'm still pissed off about it. That doctor put me through needless torture. It was extremely stupid. Not until four years later, and after two hospitalizations, was I finally diagnosed with manic-depressive illness by another doctor."

Bob Boorstin could have easily been just another tragic statistic had he not been diagnosed. An untreated brain illness leaves an individual vulnerable to grossly distorted impressions as we saw with Judge Sol Wachtler. But, bipolar disorder is also a biopsychosocial illness.

"Chemistry isn't everything," insisted Bob. "Focusing only on chemistry is mindless, but focusing solely on psychosocial influences is brainless."

Regrettably, Bob's stepfather's life was also cut short when he was killed in a freak highway accident. His death left Bob bereft. Following years of pain and turmoil, at age 37, Boorstin finally married and settled down.

> I visited the shrink four to five days each week for two years and was never diagnosed. I'm still pissed off about it. That doctor put me through needless torture. Not until four years later, and after two hospitalizations, was I finally diagnosed with manic-depressive illness by another doctor.
>
> —BOB BOORSTIN

"Ten years ago," said Bob, "had somebody predicted that today I'd be a happily married family man I would have vehemently disputed it. 'Hell no,' I would have insisted. 'It [marriage] is not for someone like me.'"

Both Nancy and Bernie experienced sorrow that anyone as gifted as Bob Boorstin could have such self-deprecating thoughts. It was not "outside" stigma that affected Bob, but "internal" shame that directed his thinking in this area.

"When my wife and I were first married," he continued, "we had planned not to have children. 'Why,' we belabored, 'bring kids into this world knowing that any offspring of ours would have a 25-percent chance of being afflicted with bipolar disorder?' That seemed irresponsible." Bob credited ego with changing his mind. "Besides, my own condition is under control and I know what to look for. We also have hope of future advances in treatment and research," he added.

When Nancy and her husband were first married in 1966, neither was aware of her bipolar condition. As she now looks back, she can see early indications of the disorder, but it would be some years before her symptoms became obvious. In fact, at that time she had no idea that manic-depression existed in her family, nor did she know what the illness was all about. Nevertheless, had Nancy been properly informed of her genetic predisposition to bipolar disorder

> Bipolar disorder is tremendously destructive to relationships. The divorce rate among marriages in which a spouse is manic-depressive is very high.

her decision regarding children would have been the same. She would not have hesitated to have children. Like Bob Boorstin, Nancy's condition is now under control and she, too, knows what to look for.

At the time this book is going to press, Dr. Frederick Goodwin has predicted that genetic vulnerability to bipolar illness will be greatly diminished within five years. "Genetic markers will be clinically available to diagnose, to treat ahead, and thereby to prevent offspring from inheriting mental illnesses such as unipolar and manic-depression," he stated during a telephone call with Nancy.

BIPOLAR DISORDER AND RELATIONSHIPS

Bipolar disorder is tremendously destructive to relationships. The divorce rate among marriages in which a spouse is manic-depressive is very high. It is demoralizing for a husband or wife to endure a day-to-day relationship with someone from whom they can't get a positive response, and who they can't help. Manic episodes can be as daunting for a partner to endure as can depressive ones. People like to believe they can contribute to their partner's getting better. "Count your blessings," a spouse will tell his mate. But while the intention is to cheer and show support, such reassurances don't work for a person with bipolar disorder. A partner cannot alter the course of the illness, and the well-meaning spouse ends up feeling rejected and frustrated. People blame themselves for not being able to turn their partner's illness around.

When a person with bipolar disorder becomes intense, the very elevation of his or her mood can frequently create problems with interpersonal relationships. Intensity can fuel powerful manifestations of ebullience, overconfidence, and volatility. These episodes may fluctuate dramatically and be interspersed with periods of irritability and rage. "We, the afflicted, become transported into a world of unlimited ideas and possibilities. The sky's the limit!" said Nancy.

> When someone whose spouse is in a manic episode and refuses treatment asks me what he or she can do, I tell them to "close the bank account and wait it out."
>
> —JAN FAWCETT

"While we're soaring, other people frequently are put off by such apparent grandiosity. We may seem too talkative, uninhibited, pompous, manipulative, or intrusive; our ideas may sound outlandish; or we may exhibit other irresponsible or inappropriate behavior. Such characteristics are manifested during periods of mania, or hypomania (less extreme), and our seemingly inexhaustible supply of energy and self-confidence can erode, and even torpedo, relationships.

"'You're not hearing me,' I've been told on numerous occasions," said Nancy. "Although I might have heard every word, at that moment I may not have been in a position to control my garrulousness. When my bipolar condition kicks in, oftentimes it's accompanied by irrational behavior. I feel distraught."

In a troubled marriage, the ill person usually gets the blame immediately and receives no support from his or her partner. But any relationship can quickly deteriorate, and even the strongest ones can be extinguished over time. Women, more often than men, are the more traditional caretakers. As a result, more women than men will stay around to nurture and support the relationship when illness strikes a loved one.

The Effects of Stress, Intensity, and Trauma

Any traumatic episode can trigger symptoms in people with bipolar disorder, which likely appear overreactive to others. While some individuals are better equipped to handle shocks than others are, the average person is not thrown completely off balance by a simple twist of fate. But in a person who has bipolar disorder, trauma produces an uncontrollable emotional upheaval, unwittingly leading to poor judgment and intrusiveness.

"I felt recently blown away by the apparent disloyalty of a former associate," said Nancy. "When it was brought to my attention that this person had dealt me yet another painful blow, I was stunned. Following the dissolution of our association that had been prompted by irreconcilable differences, I thought my troubles were over. But, the nightmare of that unhappy episode returned to haunt me like a bad movie which flashed before my eyes. I felt instantly threatened and morally violated; trapped, once again, inside a vicious web. A temporary loss of faith in all humanity had returned momentarily because of the injustice which I felt had been committed. The resulting trauma brought out the worst in me, and for 24 hours I was unable to function normally." Someone not prone to bipolar disorder might have handled this situation in a more balanced fashion without "going off the deep end" as Nancy had.

> As approval turns to contempt and friend to foe, we the afflicted find ourselves in a state of overwhelming despair. Impenetrable walls seem to spring up before our eyes, separating "us" from "them."
>
> —NANCY ROSENFELD

Trauma can create the most insurmountable form of stress—pressure so intense that it not only inflames, but also permanently damages, an existing relationship. "As approval turns to contempt and friend to foe, we the afflicted find ourselves in a state of overwhelming despair," said Nancy.

"Impenetrable walls seem to spring up before our eyes, separating 'us' from 'them.'"

Some relationships never recover from these painful, regrettable, and inopportune, shock waves. But, life is filled with endings and new beginnings. Relationships may come and go, but, no matter how fleeting they are, it is from these experiences that people gain strength and wisdom.

SUMMARY

Living, and thriving, with bipolar disorder may not be easy, but it's possible—even probable—if you are willing to accept the challenge. As with any other obstacle, even some grave misfortune, there is a bright side. Moreover, everyone has choices when confronted with challenging situations. It is the responsibility of each one of us to determine *how* to overcome our individual problems and be able to turn negatives into positives. Survivors of this disorder need to understand that they are not their illness: The afflicted *have* bipolar illness, but they are *not* bipolar disorder.

CHAPTER 2

Diagnosis of Bipolar Disorder

A DIAGNOSIS CONVEYS the cluster of symptoms that character-ize a disorder. A correct diagnosis points the way to treatments that have proven helpful. If the medical field is sufficiently advanced in the area of a particular illness, understanding of its various causes and mechanisms ultimately leads to the development of better treat-ment. With this information, the physician can design a course of treatment based on the newest and most effective therapies available.

Psychiatric disorders are manifested by emotions, thoughts, and behavior. Yet our culture, and even medical training, has erroneously separated concepts of mind from the body as if they are totally unrelated. Mood and behavior are often considered a result of self-discipline, strength of character, and moral choice for which we bear responsibility, while physical illness is considered an unfortunate event outside of one's control. The fact that the mind is controlled by and dependent on normal brain function is often denied or ignored. The result is an inability to view the manifestations of psychiatric dis-orders in the same way that medical disorders are viewed. If a person develops severe depression after a serious head injury, it is understood that a tissue injury is related to the depressive behavior. If a person develops severe depression in conjunction with bipolar disorder, the behavior may be considered a voluntary choice on the part of the patient.

WHY IS BIPOLAR DISORDER CALLED AN ILLNESS?

Although everyone experiences ups and downs—happiness, sadness, and anger are normal emotions—people with manic-depression have mood swings out of proportion, or totally unrelated, to what is going on in their lives. While the occurrence of mania or depression may follow a life stress, the pathological mood state tends to persist long after the stressful situation is resolved.

> Historically, people believed that devil possession was the cause of psychiatric disorders. While this belief has fallen out of favor, a different stigma has taken its place; today, the assumed cause is often a moral or character weakness.

A lack of good animal models for psychiatric illnesses, as well as the technical and ethical difficulties in studying human brain function are the reasons that research studies have only recently begun to collect data analyzing mood disorders. Historically, people believed that devil possession was the cause of psychiatric disorders. While this belief has fallen out of favor, a different stigma has taken its place; today, the assumed cause is often a moral or character weakness. The reality is that chemical changes in the brain and genetic factors are the real culprits.

As you may know, the original name for bipolar disorder was manic-depressive psychosis. One of the reasons for the change of terminology may well have been the stigma attached to the earlier name since people frequently mischaracterized the diagnosis as "maniac" (rather than "manic") depressive illness. This is why psychiatric diagnoses, such as bipolar disorder, are often considered "labels" (or tags). The social meaning for these illnesses is different from the medical diagnoses. These are labels that we understandably consider harmful and want to avoid but arriving at a correct diagnosis is crucial to a patient's well-being.

THE DIFFICULTY OF DIAGNOSING BIPOLAR DISORDER

Bipolar disorder can be a difficult illness to diagnose. The diagnosis may immediately subject a patient to social disapproval and shame because of its stigma. Fear and ignorance can even affect the attitude of people who might otherwise seem educated or sophisticated. Like clinical depression, bipolar disorder is frequently attributed to a weakness of character. As a result of this stigma, the details of a family history of mental illness, which would ordinarily aid in the diagnosis of bipolar disorder, may be hidden or "forgotten" by patients or relatives. This is important since accurate patient and family histories are often important in making the diagnosis.

> In general, families and friends are much more comfortable in dealing with depressive episodes rather than the manic or hypomanic stages of the illness.

Manic or hypomanic episodes can increase other people's anxiety about the disorder because of the unpredictability of behavior and lack of control that often accompany such episodes. In general, families and friends are much more comfortable in dealing with depressive episodes rather than the manic or hypomanic stages of the illness.

On the other hand, some people in hypomanic states—characterized by euphoria, optimism, and increased confidence and energy—may be very charismatic, interesting, and uplifting to be with. They sometimes exercise leadership, convince others, and make excellent salespeople of both things and ideas. These individuals rarely perceive such states as pathological, but instead tend to value the increased levels of energy, confidence, and creativity that flow during these episodes. Consequently, people in a hypomanic state may view hypomania as a normal pattern of behavior and refuse any treatment that might compromise their energy and creativity.

The diagnosis of bipolar disorder is largely based on the history of prior behaviors, thought patterns, and moods, as well as family history of mood disorders. Therefore, it is important for a clinician to actively seek this information from the patient. Even though mood swings may not be apparent initially to the patient, the nature of this pattern provides the physician with critical data for analysis.

ONSET OF BIPOLAR DISORDER

Bipolar disorder can start in early childhood, or as late as the 40s and 50s (see figure 2.1). Over age 50, the cause of an episode is more likely to be a problem that imitates bipolar disorder, such as neurological illness or the effects of drugs, alcohol, or a prescription medicine. Frequently, bipolar disorder is manifested for the first time during adolescence, which is a time of "normal" turmoil. Some people may hold the view that normal adolescence is a kind of "psychosis" in itself. Since moodiness and various crises around school and relationships often occur during the teen years, it is easy to understand how the early symptoms of bipolar disorder might first be incorrectly attributed to "normal" adolescent problems.[1] Bestselling author Danielle Steel's son Nick, to whom we refer again, is an example of a troubled youth whose bipolar illness was neither fully understood nor properly managed.

Some people in hypomanic states are very charismatic, interesting, and uplifting to be with. These individuals rarely perceive such states as pathological, but instead tend to value the increased levels of energy, confidence, and creativity that flow during these episodes.

Clinical scientists have found that the initial episodes of depression or hyperactivity, frequently attributed later to bipolar illness (when a doctor finally makes the diagnosis), occur in response to some life stress. The patient's history will clearly show subsequent

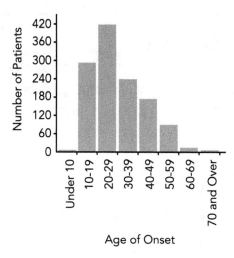

Figure 2.1. *Age of Onset of Bipolar Disorder*

(Source: *Manic-Depressive Illness* by Frederick K. Goodwin and Kay R. Jamison, copyright 1990 by Oxford University Press, Inc. Used by permission of Oxford University Press, Inc.)

episodes, which may have occurred without any identifiable life stress. The illness becomes autonomous and mood swings recur cyclically in a pattern that can be discerned in retrospect.

All too often doctors fail to arrive at an early diagnosis. People with bipolar disorder see, on an average, three to four doctors and spend more than eight years seeking treatment before receiving a correct diagnosis.

IMPORTANCE OF EARLY DIAGNOSIS

In young people, bipolar disorder can be severe enough to interfere with school. It may also cause its victim to miss the usual social and identity development associated with adolescence. Adolescent development can be distorted by episodes of depression, nonfunction, crises resulting from impulsive behaviors, bad judgments made during manic mood swings, and repeated hospitalizations. The adolescent's identity becomes that of a patient instead of a student who is building a future adult identity and career.

Early Diagnosis as Prevention

Early diagnosis, proper treatment, and finding the right medication at a young age is crucial in helping people to avoid the following destructive social and health outcomes:

- Suicide
- Alcohol/substance abuse
- Marital and work problems
- Treatment difficulties
- Incorrect, inappropriate, or partial treatment

The additional problems of alcohol and substance abuse, which are hazards for any young person today, are common with bipolar disorder. This is called a "comorbid" condition. Rates of alcohol and substance abuse comorbidity of 50 to 70 percent have been reported associated with bipolar disorder. The two illnesses augment each other in their power to damage or even destroy a young life. This happened to Nick Traina when he began to abuse over-the-counter medications at the age of 11 to "still the demons." Comorbidity finally killed him.

In young people, bipolar disorder can cause its victim to miss the usual social and identity development associated with adolescence.

Family education leads to early diagnosis and treatment, resulting in "harm reduction." An early response may help reduce or prevent the negative impact of bipolar disorder on life—social impairment, school failure, legal problems, hospitalizations, and others. A family history of bipolar disorder may be present, providing a strong clue for the family and clinician. As mentioned above, however, family shame and denial may hide this history, making early recognition more difficult. In addition, as will be discussed later, adult individuals with bipolar disorder may function at high levels despite their disorder, thus further obscuring the diagnosis and the establishment of a family history.

Some of these patients have a mild form of the illness known as cyclothymia (see page 44). This is characterized by depressive periods lasting weeks or months and then mild hypomanic periods during which the person experiences increased energy, mental alertness, confidence, and decreased need for sleep that may make considerable success attainable. Many people with a history of depression and hypomania do not seek treatment for several years. In fact, these individuals may be quite creative and successful in their careers.

SYMPTOMS OF BIPOLAR DISORDER

We have alluded to various types of bipolar disorder above. The variation in symptoms and in the severity of the illness in different individuals is one reason for the difficulty in obtaining a proper diagnosis. Even trained specialists in psychiatry might miss the diagnosis when it presents in certain atypical forms.

> The variation in symptoms and in the severity of bipolar disorder in different individuals is one reason for the difficulty in obtaining a proper diagnosis.

Mania, hypomania, and depression are the general categories of symptoms involved in bipolar disorder. Bipolar disorder differs significantly from clinical depression. In bipolar disorder, a person's mood alternates between mania and depression. One swing of the mood pendulum can last for days, weeks, or even months, or in other instances moods may change rapidly alternating with normal periods. It is important to inform your physician of all mood swings, past or present, so a correct diagnosis can be made.

Mania

Mania often begins with a pleasurable sense of heightened energy, creativity, and social ease. People with mania lack insight, deny anything is wrong, and angrily blame others for pointing out a problem. In a manic state, some or all of the following symptoms are present for at least one week, and the person has trouble functioning in a normal way:

- Heightened mood and exaggerated optimism and self-confidence
- Decreased need for sleep, without fatigue
- Grandiose delusions, inflated sense of self-importance
- Excessive irritability, aggressive behavior
- Increased physical and mental activity
- Rapid, pressured speech, flight of ideas from one topic to another, distractability
- Poor judgment, impulsiveness
- Reckless behavior such as spending sprees, rash business decisions, erratic driving, sexual indiscretions

Anyone experiencing some of these symptoms, which often alternate with symptoms of depression (below), should seek help from a medical professional if the symptoms persist for several days and cannot be attributed to drug or alcohol abuse.

Hypomania

A milder form of mania, hypomania has similar but less severe symptoms and impairment. It is characterized by increased energy, increased activity, decreased need for sleep, increased confidence, sexual drive, poor judgment, impulsive behavior, euphoria or irritability, and sometimes grandiosity, but without psychosis. Friends and relatives notice that the behavior is not usual for the individual. Psychoses (e.g., delusions of having special powers) is not present in hypomania, but is present in mania in about 50 percent of cases.

Depression

Major depression is characterized by five or more of the following symptoms, lasting for at least two weeks and making it difficult to function:

- Depressed mood most of the day or markedly diminished interest or pleasure in all or almost all activities for most of the day
- Significant changes in appetite or sleep patterns
- Loss of enjoyment or pleasure in usual activities
- Loss of motivation
- Loss of energy, persistent lethargy
- Feelings of guilt and worthlessness
- Inability to concentrate, indecisiveness
- Slowing of speech, thought, and body movement
- Physical agitation and restlessness
- Recurring thoughts of death or suicide

In addition, although not criterion symptoms for the diagnosis, patients with major depression frequently show irritability, anger, worry, agitation, anxiety, and physical symptoms such as various types of pain and nausea. If you have thoughts of death or suicide, tell a medical professional, friend, or a member of the clergy *immediately*.

DIFFERENT PATTERNS OF BIPOLAR DISORDER

There is a spectrum of symptom severity in bipolar disorder that can obscure the diagnosis, as discussed above. There are also subtypes of the disorder that can confuse the picture. These subtypes may also require different treatment, which makes it additionally important to arrive at a correct diagnosis. Reflecting the range of bipolar disorder,

Bipolar Diagnoses

- Bipolar I disorder
- Schizoaffective disorder, bipolar type
- Bipolar II disorder
- Bipolar disorder NOS (not otherwise specified)
- Cyclothymia

Subtypes of Bipolar Disorder

- Rapid-cycling bipolar disorder
- Mixed or dysphoric mania
- Bipolar spectrum disorders
- Covert cycling
- Depressive disorders

the official classification guide for diagnoses, *DSM-IV (Diagnostic and Statistical Manual, Fourth Edition)*, recognizes bipolar I disorder; schizoaffective disorder, bipolar type; bipolar II disorder; bipolar disorder NOS (not otherwise specified); and cyclothymia. Mood disorders due to an organic condition (brain tumor, subclinical stroke, traumatic brain injury, or metabolic disease) or a substance-induced mood disorder (street drugs, alcohol, and certain prescribed medications) can create symptoms that resemble bipolar disorder.

Some people have equal numbers of manic and depressive episodes. Others have mostly one type or another. The average person with bipolar disorder experiences four episodes during the first ten years of the illness. Men are more likely to start with a manic episode, women with a depressive one. Cycles vary in duration, intensity, and frequency. Some people recover completely between

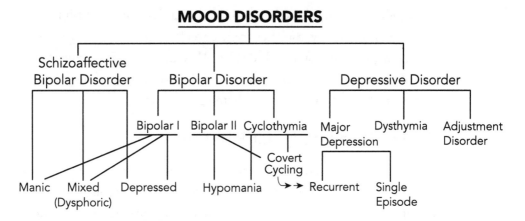

Figure 2.2. *Bipolar Mood Disorders*

episodes, but others continue to experience low-grade but troubling depression or mild mood swings.

Bipolar I Disorder

Bipolar I disorder is the most severe form of bipolar disorder, a condition that includes symptoms of hyperactivity progressing in some patients to agitation, irritability, paranoia, grandiosity, and even progressing to a delusional psychosis (characterized by an inability to appreciate reality). Additionally, patients may exhibit a progressive degree of grandiose delusions, pressured speech, distractibility, and flight of thoughts (the patient goes from one topic to another cued by words that trigger some other thought).

A high percentage of patients have severe enough symptoms to not only require medication, but also further treatment (usually hospitalization). Approximately 50 percent of patients with bipolar I disorder manifest a psychosis (the inability to distinguish reality from fantasy or belief). These patients' frequently manifest

> The average person with bipolar disorder experiences four episodes during the first ten years of the illness. Men are more likely to start with a manic episode, women with a depressive one.

poor judgment, impulsive behavior, and total lack of insight into their illness. Consequently, they may refuse treatment.

In chapter one you met Judge Sol Wachtler, who is a prime example of someone who lives with bipolar I disorder. Wachtler's bizarre behavior was responsible for his being sent to prison.

Schizoaffective Bipolar Disorder

This is another severe form of illness, considered by many to be one form of bipolar disorder, with characteristics of schizophrenia. These patients may manifest depression, mania, and persistent psychotic symptoms (hallucinations or delusions) that overlap with episodes of depression and mania and that persist beyond mood episodes. Differentiating bipolar disorder and schizophrenia can be a diagnostic challenge. (See figure 2.2.)

The differentiation between these two disorders is also a controversial subject, and one that is met with considerable confusion. Are these patients who have psychotic symptoms schizophrenic? Or manic? Or, do they suffer from severe depression with psychotic symptoms? The term schizoaffective disorder was created as a separate diagnostic category, a hybrid type of mood disorder that overlaps the criteria for schizophrenia and bipolar I disorder. But there is some evidence to indicate that schizomanic conditions are more prevalent than schizodepressive ones.[2]

> There are three stages of mania, essentially differentiated by the severity of the illness and manifested by an increasing amount of agitation and psychosis.

What is important to note is that mood-stabilizing drugs will help patients with schizoaffective bipolar disorder whereas mood stabilizers are not generally helpful in patients suffering from schizophrenia.

There are three stages of mania, essentially differentiated by the severity of the illness and manifested by an increasing amount of agitation and psychosis. Acute symptoms of irritability, anger, paranoia, and catatonic-like excitement cannot differentiate mania from schizophrenia. In a severe episode, it may be difficult to differentiate bipolar disorder from acute schizophrenia without any prior personal history and family history. Therefore, it is understandable why some research clinicians suggest that schizoaffective bipolar disorder is really a severe form of bipolar I disorder, namely that families of patients with this diagnosis have histories of bipolar disorder, not schizophrenia.

Bipolar II Disorder

The diagnosis of bipolar II disorder is frequently missed due to its subtleties. It is characterized by episodes of hypomania alternating with even longer periods of major depression that can be very severe and threatening. Although these people exhibit symptoms that are commonly recognized as "abnormal" by either the patients or their families, their symptoms are generally not severe enough to mandate hospitalization, even though there may be some interference in their normal level of functioning. However, these patients do not manifest psychosis and may not even recognize, or report, their symptoms of hypomania, choosing only to remember their depressive episodes.

Individuals with bipolar II disorder are usually the ones to seek treatment for depression and give histories of recurrent depressive episodes. They may, however, resist treatment for their disorder by electing not to take mood stabilizers, such as lithium, which tend to suppress the hypomanic periods that patients commonly associate with happiness or increased function and creativity.

Many of these patients go undiagnosed because they are treated for depression with antidepressant medications alone. This can actually increase their mood cycles and lead to recurrences of depression, rapid cycling, or the occurrence of mixed states. Doctors may misdiagnose bipolar II disorder as a severe personality disorder.

Nancy's bipolar condition seems to be in the category of bipolar II disorder. Though she once contemplated suicide and has sought therapeutic counseling, Nancy was never hospitalized for her condition. She reports that her highs and lows have been extreme. With proper management of her illness (which includes a daily maintenance program of antidepressant medication), however, Nancy functions at a high level, with minimum occurrence of mild depression.

Bipolar Disorder NOS

Bipolar disorder NOS (not otherwise specified) includes disorders with bipolar features that do not meet specific criteria for other diagnoses of bipolar disorder. Examples might be rapid alterations of mood over a period of time that does not meet the duration criteria for other diagnoses, or recurrent hypomanic episodes in the absence of depression.

Cyclothymia

Cyclothymia is the mildest form of bipolar disorder. Many patients with cyclothymia never seek diagnosis or treatment. They may function well, with some interruption during periods of mild or moderate depression alternating with mild hypomania and increased activity. These individuals can become more severely ill to the point of impairment in response to certain substances or medications (including marijuana, alcohol, antidepressants, steroids, and, possibly, high doses of decongestants), which may increase the severity of their depression or precipitate full-blown mania.

Rapid-Cycling Bipolar Disorder

Patients are arbitrarily defined as having a rapid-cycling form of bipolar I disorder or bipolar II disorder if they have four or more episodes of mania or depression in one year, in any combination. Rapid cycling also implies an increased frequency of depressive or manic episodes with shorter times of normal mood between episodes. Between 5 and 15 percent of patients with bipolar disorder fall into this category at some time in their course of illness. Patients can manifest mood cycling to the point of showing mood changes in the same day, or even within an hour. This may be termed ultra-rapid cycling (ultradian cycling).

The significance of these variations in rapid cycling is that they can lead to misdiagnosis of personality disorder or schizophrenia, which makes the condition even more difficult to treat effectively. Rapid cycling is a temporary phase of bipolar disorder that some patients, particularly women, are prone to, whereas bipolar disorder usually affects both sexes equally. Some bipolar patients go through rapid cycling for months, during which their symptoms are more difficult to control. At this time, the exact causes of rapid cycling remain unknown and there is no preventable treatment. Rapid cycling may occur at some point in a bipolar disorder and then revert to a previous pattern of an episode or two each year, depending on treatment response. Although the issue is debated, there is evidence suggesting that antidepressant agents can precipitate rapid cycling or mania in bipolar patients.

Goodwin and Jamison reported that rapid cycling is of considerable importance both theoretically and practically. From a theoretical standpoint, rapid-cycling patients make up a disproportionate percentage of the total number of cases studied. Practically speaking, the treatment of patients with rapid cycling may be different from the treatment prescribed for patients with normal cycling patterns.[3] We discuss this further in chapter 4.

Mixed or Dysphoric Mania

This is the most disabling subform of bipolar disorder because symptoms of both mania and depression occur simultaneously, or alternate frequently during the same day. The person becomes excitable and agitated as in mania, but also irritable and depressed—feeling anxiety, instead of the euphoria classically associated with mania.

This form of the illness can be found in either bipolar I disorder or bipolar II disorder. Mixed mania occurs in about 40 to 45 percent of bipolar cases. The patient presents with the restlessness, hyperactivity, irritability, and sometimes paranoia or mania, combined with symptoms of depression and distress. Missing is the positive mood or euphoric optimism of classic mania or hypomania.

> Mixed mania is the most disabling subform of bipolar disorder because symptoms of both mania and depression occur simultaneously, or alternate frequently during the day.

Doctors may mistakenly diagnose the patient as having a schizophrenic psychosis with agitation, or a paranoid state. Doctors can miss the bipolar disorder diagnosis with milder forms as well, and erroneously diagnose the condition as a severe personality disorder or substance-abuse disorder.

These patients are often more impulsive and suicidal than those who experience the other forms of bipolar disorder. They often are not capable of being cooperative in a relationship, may have a very low tolerance for stress, and frequently express anger or rage. These symptoms can be the manifestation of mixed manic states (mania and depression) or rapid cycling, both of which can occur in patients with bipolar I or bipolar II disorder.

Bipolar Spectrum Disorder

The term bipolar spectrum disorder is often used to describe a class of disorders that have bipolar features, such as recurrent mood changes associated with increased activity, impulsive behavior, and irritability alternating with depressed or dysphoric mood. This term overlaps with the bipolar NOS diagnosis in many instances.

Covert Cycling

Another form of bipolar spectrum disorder, covert cycling may not technically meet the formal criteria for bipolar disorder I or II, but may meet NOS (not otherwise specified) criteria. It is found in some proportion of patients who have a series of recurrences of depression following several months of antidepressant response to treatment.

Frequently, the patient improves with the use of another antidepressant medication only to relapse once again.

If you look carefully and talk with loved ones who know the patient well, in some cases, you may detect a pattern of hyperthymia (periods of mildly elevated mood and increased energy that seem within a normal range). This pattern is often associated with increased as well as productive activity. Patients and those around them might consider the slight mood elevation positive (an "admirable quality"), rather than viewing it as a pathological mania. The hyperthymia in these individuals is then followed by a depressive recurrence despite any maintenance program of antidepressant medication.

In covert cycling, a mood-stabilization drug added to antidepressant treatment may prevent the recurrences that happen with maintenance antidepressant treatment alone. Antidepressant medication will not prevent a depression once a hypomanic or hyperthymic mood shift has oc-

> In almost all cases of bipolar disorder, a depression follows a manic mood swing, so it is difficult, or impossible, to avoid the depressions while permitting the manic or hypomanic symptoms.

curred. In fact, in almost all cases of bipolar disorder, a depression follows a manic mood swing, so it is difficult, or impossible, to avoid the depressions while permitting the manic or hypomanic symptoms. Once patients with cyclothymia or bipolar II disorder understand this, they are more likely to accept mood-stabilization treatment.

Depressive Disorders

In sharp contrast to mania, depressive disorders are usually defined by a slowing down of almost all aspects of emotion and behavior, that is, rate of thought and speech, energy, sexuality, and the ability to experience pleasure. As with mania, the severity of depressive disorders varies widely.[4] The majority of bipolar patients experience more time in depressive states than in mania or hypomania.

At the most severe end of the spectrum is *major depression*; episodes can be recurrent or occur as a single episode. Chronic depression, or *dysthymia*, is a lingering form of mild depression (limited to two to three symptoms) that persists at least two years. Patients may not fully recover from a chronic depressive episode without treatment, and remain generally lacking in energy with a negative outlook on life. *Adjustment disorder*, the mildest form of depression, is manifested by depressive symptoms emerging under situational stress and may manifest some impairment in social or occupational function. Any impairment is generally short-lived, however, and less pervasive than a major form of depression.

SUMMARY

Doctors can fail to diagnose bipolar disorder due to the frequent difficulty of obtaining an accurate history along with the multiple levels of severity and various forms in which the illness presents. The establishment of an accurate diagnosis is important because the untreated illness can be disabling, and even dangerous, to the patient. Given that fact and the effective treatments available to us today, early diagnosis is extremely important.

Early diagnosis and treatment can restore and even save lives. People who had lost a sense of meaning and joy in life can rediscover it and return to leading a productive existence. Early diagnosis and treatment can also save careers, not to mention marriages, and reduce family strife.

CHAPTER 3

The Biology of Bipolar Disorder

Humans have a natural desire to understand the causes of human affliction and explain a disorder that manifests as emotional pain, adverse behaviors, and, in some cases, irrational thought. The causes we attribute bipolar disorder to are highly related to the predominant thought of the time as well as the degree to which scientific knowledge has developed.

WHAT CAUSES BIPOLAR DISORDER?

Bipolar disorder often stems from a genetic vulnerability that can run in families. Thus far we have evidence that the interaction of a genetic vulnerability with everyday life stresses triggers the onset of symptoms that over time seem to recur with or without specific stressful events.

Researchers have identified a number of genes that may be linked to the disorder. If you have bipolar and your spouse does not, there is a 7.8 percent risk of an offspring developing bipolar disorder and an additional 11.2 percent chance for the development of unipolar major depression, for a total risk of a mood disorder of 19 percent. The chances may be somewhat greater if a number of your relatives are afflicted with the disorder, or if the onset of the disorder was in childhood or adolescence. If both parents have a history of bipolar disorder, there is a 50 to 75 percent chance of their child developing a mood disorder. Note that the chances of an offspring developing unipolar major depression are greater than the chances of developing of a bipolar disorder. Recent epidemiological studies have determined that just over 1 percent of the population has symptoms of various forms of bipolar disorder.

Epidemiological evidence can chart the scope of an illness, its likely course, likely associated or comorbid conditions (such as anxiety or alcohol abuse disorders), and possible risk factors. In addition, these studies are used to link the occurrence of the illness with genetic, psychological, social, and environmental factors. This data can also be effective in planning research into the causes of the illness as well as designing treatment or even preventive programs.

> Bipolar disorder often stems from a genetic vulnerability that can run in families. Thus far, we have evidence that the interaction of a genetic vulnerability with everyday life stresses triggers the onset of symptoms which over time seem to recur autonomously with or without specific stressful events.

In this chapter, we will review some of the large and rapidly growing bodies of evidence from family studies, as well as imaging neurochemical, and pharmacologic studies, that convey what we know and what we are rapidly learning about the psychobiology of bipolar disorder. This area is progressing rapidly, and varying newly developed methods are being utilized. Therefore, findings may not be in agreement until more research has been done. While the new is not always the ultimate truth, one has to view the emerging findings in the perspective of the past. This chapter will try to summarize those directions and emerging findings in the biology of bipolar disorder.

While groundbreaking studies establishing a new method of treatment of mood disorders such as bipolar disorder and major depression or even introducing a new treatment paradigm (e.g., the 1970 introduction in this country of lithium as a treatment for bipolar disorder) occasionally emerge, the majority of these scientific findings advance our knowledge in small increments. Sometimes new discoveries reverse, or even redirect, former ways of thinking. Scientific progress originates from this sea of findings. It is the product of a mass of research efforts, one adding to another. With this caveat, we will attempt to summarize some areas of research into the psychobiology of bipolar disorder.

PSYCHOBIOLOGICAL FINDINGS

As knowledge has grown concerning the possible causes of bipolar disorder and related affective disorders, it has become clear that biological factors are at least necessary, if not sufficient, conditions for their occurrence.

Goodwin and Jamison's *Manic Depressive Illness* presents evidence of contributing biological factors to the development of bipolar disorder, from the earliest recorded studies to 1990, offering summary statements to guide us. Summary statements from this book offer the challenge that any set of findings purporting to be relevant to the causes of manic-depressive illness (bipolar disorder) must account for both genetic vulnerability and the cyclical (recurrent) nature of the illness. Its cyclical nature means that it has the tendency to recur, and without adequate treatment will certainly recur over time.

> As knowledge has grown concerning the possible causes of bipolar disorder and related disorders, it has become clear that biological factors are at least necessary, if not sufficient, conditions for their occurrence.

Findings of genetic vulnerability are the cornerstones of efforts to explain the causes of bipolar disorder. Attempting to account for the cyclical nature of this illness has been difficult to study at the biological level because few, if any, suitable animal models of bipolar disorder exist. Animal studies permit the use of certain invasive scientific methods that cannot be used in humans. These studies have been a major source of progress in our understanding of cancer, infectious diseases, heart disease, and other illnesses. Because illnesses such as bipolar disorder manifest themselves in behaviors specific to humans, we are limited in applying these animal models the way we can utilize them to understand other human illnesses.

Initial research focused on genetic vulnerability as the cause of bipolar disorder. Later, as a result of observing the effect of medications such as lithium and antidepressants on the course of the illness, scientists began to consider the contribution of alterations in brain chemicals called neurotransmitters. Dr. Lewis Opler explained in layperson's terms how these chemicals work: "We have nerve cells in our brain that are separated by tiny little spaces called 'synapses.' Chemicals called 'neurotransmitters' send messages across these spaces, and these messages signal our brain to do its job. Neurotransmitters come in all different sizes, and these chemicals fit neatly into 'receptors' that are located on the surfaces of other cells."[1] Recent research is focusing on the chemical reactions initiated within the nerve cell by these receptors and their effect on releasing complex chemical messengers within the cells, as well as the activation of certain genes.

GENETIC PREDISPOSITION TO BIPOLAR DISORDER

Scientifically based evidence supports the theory of genetic predisposition to bipolar disorder. Let's examine recent findings that support this correlation. Dr. Elliot S. Gershon summarizes the most powerful evidence of genetic vulnerability to bipolar illness. He points out that the strongest evidence comes from studies of identical (monozygotic or MZ) twins compared with fraternal (dizygotic or DZ) twins. The MZ twins share identical genes and environment, while DZ twins share a similar environment, but have a slightly different genetic makeup.[2]

In these studies, the concordance rate, or rate of similarity (meaning both twins had affective illness), was from 62 to 72 percent (with an additional 18 to 25 percent with unipolar depression) for the MZ twins and 0 to 8 percent (with an additional 0 to 11 percent with unipolar depression) for the DZ twins.

In a more recent psychiatric review of twin studies, Norwegian psychiatrist E. Kringlen reported his observations on the relatively strong contribution genetics makes to Alzheimer's disease, bipolar disorder, schizophrenia, and childhood autism. Since the concordance rates are far from 100 percent in most of these illnesses, environmental factors must also be important.[3] This observation is important in light of increasing neurobiological research showing that experience can modify biochemical processes in the brain to a degree not previously appreciated. The implications of such "brain plasticity" will be discussed later.

Additional genetic evidence is found in adoption studies, a research method most frequently used in Scandinavian countries. Two studies of children whose biological parents also had bipolar disorder, but who were adopted when less than 6 months of age and raised by non-bipolar adoptive parents, have provided support for the involvement of genetic factors in familial transmission.[4]

Data from over 40 studies has revealed that the risk for bipolar disorder is consistently higher for relatives of those with the disorder than it is for relatives of normal controls. The risk for both bipolar and unipolar disorders is higher in the relatives of bipolar subjects, whereas the first-degree relatives of unipolar depression subjects have a higher rate of unipolar depression alone.[5] We can conclude that affective disorders are familial as a result of genetic transmission, and the most frequent affective disorder among relatives of bipolar patients is unipolar depression, not bipolar disorder.

In families where there is evidence of early onset (childhood or adolescent) bipolar disorder, the likelihood that another family member will be affected by the disorder is above the average for affected families overall. Moreover, the more severe forms of bipolar or

Genetic Vulnerabilities

Summarizing the studies of genetic factors in the transmission of vulnerability suggests the following conclusions:

1. Affective disorders run in families and this is due to a genetic vulnerability.

2. Unipolar depression is the most frequent affective disorder in relatives of bipolar patients; bipolar disorder ranks second.

3. Bipolar disorder tends to strike more frequently among relatives of unipolar patients than in control groups.

4. The likelihood of familial manifestations of affective disorders is more commonly associated with both early onset and the severity of the illness.

schizoaffective bipolar disorder, such as those with psychosis or rapid recurrences, seem to confer greater risk of the illness appearing in another family member than the usual risk for affected families.

This review of the scientific literature also demonstrates that in bipolar disorder the mode of inheritance is complex and likely involves multiple interacting genes.[6]

Cohort Effect

Some epidemiological studies have shown what is called a "cohort effect," an increased incidence, in both bipolar and unipolar depression, beginning in the 1930s and appearing to spiral upward thereafter. The cohort effect cannot be attributed to genetic alteration because it occurred over too short a period of time. Instead, it must reflect a cultural influence on expression of vulnerability to the disorders. This suggests that genetic vulnerability may be necessary but, without certain stress factors, insufficient for the expression of an illness, similar to Kringlin's observation concerning incomplete concordance in identical twins (see above).

We might ask ourselves just what in our culture is producing the increased incidence of these mental disorders. Is it our ever higher, often unmet, materialistic expectations? Or is it the greater informational load from early age as a result of television and other media? Or, perhaps, could the problem stem from dietary changes such as a decrease in omega-3 fatty acids? It has been asserted that changes in agribusiness have reduced the sources of these important dietary constituents, which make up a good part of our central nervous system and which our bodies cannot produce. Fish, fish oil, and flaxseed oil are our remaining sources of these essential fatty acids. It has been reported that while cattle once fed principally on plants containing omega-3 fatty acids, special feeds that exclude these nutrients are now principally used. These vital substances are not presently included in infant formula (but are highly concentrated in human breast milk).

Some investigators have found that the incidence of both bipolar and unipolar depression has been increasing, beginning in the 1930s and spiraling thereafter. Such an increase cannot be attributed to genetic alteration because it occurred over too short a period of time. We might ask ourselves just what in our culture is producing the increased incidence of these mental disorders.

The Harvard School of Public Health Study, conducted by Murray and associates for the World Bank, found that clinical depression is presently the world's fourth most frequent cause of disability; bipolar disorder is the sixth cause of disability. This data takes all possible causes of disability into account, from war and malnutrition to every known disease of humankind. Moreover, the study predicted that by 2020 clinical depression will be the world's second most common cause of disability.[7]

It appears that depressive illness becomes a more frequent and severe problem as populations become more technologically advanced. This could be secondary to the rate of change, and increased competition and level of expectations (both for increased material wealth and performance requirements) resulting from technological progress.

Medical scientists can only make observations concerning genetic transmission, and then it becomes necessary to study ways of reducing biological vulnerability to life stress and to develop coping techniques (see chapter 7, "Stigma," and chapter 8, "Optimism, Hope, and Transcendence").

Molecular Genetics

Rapid progress from powerful methods in molecular genetics, a relatively new field, has led to findings of "markers" for genes associated with bipolar disorders at a specific area on various genes. Technological advances have increased the capacity to scan for these markers. Progress in molecular genetics has in little more than 15 years leaped from looking for markers for genes associated with bipolar illness to looking for candidate genes that produce various substances which regulate neurochemical reactions in the brain that result in symptoms of bipolar disorder.

Chromosomal Linkage

Studies have identified regions of interest in linkage studies (establishing linkage between a certain location on a chromosome from affected individuals as compared with unaffected relatives) on chromosomes 4, 8, 10, 12, 16, 18, and 21, and the X chromosome of the human genome. Research is currently looking at genes that code for receptors, reuptake transporters (these control the metabolism of neurotransmitters in the brain by regulating the rate at which they are taken back into the nerve ending for breakdown or restorage), or critical neurotransmitters known to be affected by medications that improve the course of bipolar disorder (lithium and antidepressants). Improved techniques increase the likelihood that scientists will identify critical mechanisms in the expression of the symptoms of bipolar disorder.

INSIDE THE HUMAN BRAIN

The human brain is a highly complex structure and is located at the upper end of the *spinal cord* (see figure 3.1). In its overall appearance, the brain is a large agglomeration of delicate nerve cells and crisscrossing nerve pathways. An average adult brain weighs about 3½ pounds (no larger than a grapefruit), and is molded into two symmetrical halves or *hemispheres*. This bulbous structure of gray and white matter consists of approximately 100 billion nerve cells, or neurons, and blood vessels. Neurons consisting of a cell body and fibers are held together and connected by the fibers. Gray matter is composed of nerve cells and their surrounding mesh of fibers.

The *cerebral cortex* is the largest section of the human brain and is about 85 percent of its weight. This section consists of the right and left hemispheres and is covered by a thin carpet of gray matter. It is

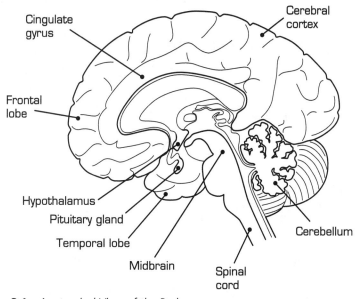

Figure 3.1—*Anatomical View of the Brain*

the cerebral cortex that controls our mental processes such as memory, speech, and thought.

The two hemispheres of the cerebral cortex are divided into lobes—*frontal* and *prefrontal, temporal, parietal,* and *occipital.* The frontal and prefrontal lobes are located behind the forehead, which appears to be the center of human intelligence, refined emotions , and one's individual personality. Most important, the prefrontal lobe controls our ability to plan functions and to initiate thought and memory.

Deep in the temporal lobe is an almond-shaped center called the *amygdala* (see figure 3.2). The amygdala (and *hippocampus,* an underlying cortical structure) controls memory and determines emotional reactions such as elation, excitement, anxiety, agitation, rage, and aggression. It also regulates the capacity to start and stop behaviors associated with these emotions. The *cingulate gyrus* is a convoluted portion of the cortex that conducts many limbic system fibers.

Beneath the cortex is white matter containing nerve cells that connect the cortex with the brain stem, and one area of the cortex with another. Groups of nerve cells called the *basal ganglia* lie deeply below the cortex.

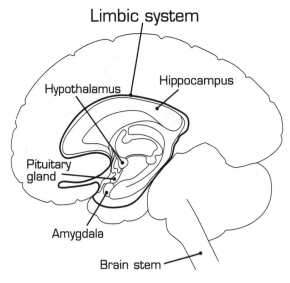

Figure 3.2—*Limbic System*

The *hypothalamus* is a cluster of cells, and at 4 grams it is the size of a walnut. This governs the sex drive (or libido), regulates body temperature, controls appetite and sleep patterns, and is responsible for mood changes and emotions such as fear and rage. The hypothalamus also controls the pituitary gland. The *pituitary gland* is a major endocrine gland located at the base of the brain. Its hormones regulate growth and control the secretions of other endocrine glands, such as the thyroid and adrenals. But, what is important to note is that the pituitary gland regulates the hormonal stress responses of the body, which have a direct effect on brain function as well.

The *midbrain* is the area on which most affective disorder researchers focus. The midbrain is an origin of neurons that produce chemicals such as serotonin and norepinephrine. These chemicals are highly important in mood disorders. Nerve impulses are activated

> It is believed that depression is associated with a reduction of serotonin or norepinephrine transmitters. Conversely, a rapid increase of these chemicals may trigger mania.

and carried from one brain cell to another by the sum total of neurotransmitters released. It is believed that there are numerous neurotransmitters, many of which are not yet known. It is further believed that depression is associated with a reduction of serotonin or norepinephrine transmitters. Conversely, a rapid increase of these chemicals may trigger mania. We will discuss this further in chapter 4.

The lower part of the brain is called the *cerebellum*. Situated beneath the cerebral cortex, the cerebellum controls muscle coordination, whereas the cerebral cortex controls our conscious thoughts and actions.

BEHAVIOR AND BIOLOGY AS TREATMENT TARGETS

We have stressed the importance of making an accurate diagnosis of bipolar disorder so that proper treatment can be initiated as early as possible to avoid the cumulative damage this illness can cause if left untreated. This section, which deals with some recent scientific advances, may at first seem to contradict this position. Early diagnosis and treatment will always remain a priority. But, as we review the findings of a wide variety of studies, new understandings relevant to the treatment of bipolar disorder and related depression may emerge.

For instance, we have discussed the fact that various subforms of bipolar disorder (e.g., rapid cycling, mixed or dysphoric states) may be more effectively treated by one medication or another that better suppresses symptoms of that form of the illness. Studies have indicated that divalproex (Depakote) maybe particularly helpful in addressing mixed states of bipolar disorder, while lithium may be more useful to address depression and the long-term risk of suicide.

Both biological findings and the results of various treatment studies are beginning to point to the importance of behavioral dimensions of bipolar and other disorders. We will be considering this point as we review findings from this perspective of some overlap between genetic studies of bipolar disorder and schizophrenia.

Research has revealed overlap between schizophrenia and bipolar disorder in three regions on chromosomes 13, 18, and 22 of the genome. This raises the possibility that schizophrenia and bipolar disorder share some susceptibility factors. This is supported by the findings of family studies that first-degree relatives of bipolar and schizophrenic patients are at increased risk for both schizoaffective disorder (symptoms of both bipolar disorder and schizophrenia) and recurrent unipolar depression.

Oligogenic Inheritance

Dr. Elliot Gershon points out that oligogenic inheritance, inheritance due to several genes, of most diseases has frustrated efforts to establish linkages based on an assumption of single gene inheritance (see figure 3.3).[8] This figure illustrates that it may require the occurrence of three or more susceptibility genes to produce a vulnerability. More advanced approaches taking oligogenic inheritance into account should lead to further progress in genetic research in bipolar and

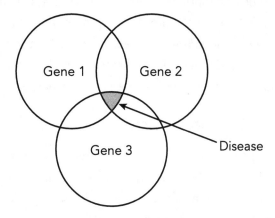

Figure 3.3—*Oligogenic Inheritance*

other disorders. As mentioned earlier, genetic research has gone be-yond merely establishing a connection between markers for genes and bipolar disorder. The goal now is to isolate the genes, identify the proteins they code, and then determine the processes they activate that lead to the emergence of symptoms in bipolar disorder. Finding new ways to block the expression of identified "bipolar symptom component" genes could prevent the emergence of the symptoms of bipolar and other affective disorders.

It may take hundreds of studies or further breakthroughs in method to reach this point. Even then, researchers may find that the genetic vulnerabilities for these disorders are different in people from different ethnic or genetic backgrounds. The multiple-gene nature of illness vulnerability adds to the complexity of the search for answers.

It is possible that affective disorders are like fevers, with similar symptoms caused by different disease processes or vulnerabilities. Successful efforts to decode the human genome have already led to the identification of cancers with the same apparent cell type (but which can be differentiated on the basis on molecular-genetic studies) that have very different treatment responses. This same approach may identify types of bipolar disorder that respond to different medications despite identical clinical symptoms and clinical diagnosis. In short, genetic research holds great promise for the future, but the direct benefits and practical applications in diagnosis, treatment, and prevention are likely to take some time to emerge.

Studies of Neurotransmitters

Research into various neurotransmitters, the enzymes involved in their synthesis and breakdown, and the receptors they activate or inhibit is an outgrowth of the "Psychopharmacologic Revolution" that started in the United States in the 1960s.

This revolution began with three developments in the area of medication: the success of chlorpromazine (Thorazine) in blocking symptoms of delusions and hallucinations, principally in schizophrenia, but also in bipolar disorder; the discovery that imipramine (Tofranil) can reverse symptoms of severe depression; and the ability of a simple salt mined from the earth—lithium—to reduce symptoms of mania and prevent recurrences of mania and depression.

These therapeutic advances literally caused a paradigm shift in the treatment of severe mental illness. In the early 1950s, prior to the introduction of chlorpromazine, the population in state hospitals was increasing at the rate of 10 percent a year. With no treatment other than restraints and crudely administered electroconvulsive therapy (ECT), these state hospitals resembled the "snake pit" mental institutions so vividly portrayed in the movies *The Snake Pit* and *One Flew Over the Cuckoo's Nest*.

After the introduction of antipsychotic medications, these populations decreased by 10 percent a year, as more patients could be discharged and fewer required admission and long-term (sometimes lifetime) hospital stays. Unfortunately, this success prompted policy makers to close state hospitals without sufficient assurances of supportive services and continued treatment as outpatients in the community. The result has been the expansion of the ranks of mentally ill homeless individuals we see on the streets of our cities today and county jails becoming the repository for acutely mentally ill persons without access to proper treatment.

Mechanisms of Drug Actions

The effects of chlorpromazine, imipramine, and lithium on mental disorders resulted in a torrent of basic laboratory studies and human clinical studies of the mechanism of action of these medications. The resulting information led to the formulation of biochemical theories, which in turn led to more knowledge about the neurotransmitter and receptor changes underlying bipolar disorders, depressive disorders, and schizophrenia. Research focused on three major brain neurotransmitters: serotonin, related to depression, mood stability, and aggression/impulsivity; dopamine, related to schizophrenia, psychosis, and mania; and norepinephrine, related to depression. Further research led to the development of medications that behave like these neurotransmitters in that they affect similar systems in the brain. A major obstacle to achieving a more complete understanding of how these neurotransmitters and their receptors, and second messenger systems within the nerve cell activated by receptors, are altered in illness such as bipolar disorder is the limitations on study of their function in the living human brain. The brain has a functional barrier that selects various biochemicals in the blood and controls their rate of passage in and out of the brain. This blood-brain barrier results in the brain maintaining a certain "metabolic independence" even though it depends on the body for nourishment and life. The significance of this in terms of research is that the blood-brain barrier limits any simple generalizations about brain function based on samples of easily obtainable body fluids such as blood.

Diseases such as hypertension, diabetes, and cancer can be more readily studied in animals where organs can be probed after such conditions are created in the animal. Scientists have so far not found any animal models of bipolar disorder. The closest approximation has been the "kindling" model, which induces spontaneous seizures by repeated electrical stimulation of the brain. While it may present a good analogy for bipolar and recurrent mood disorder as a model of a recurrent disorder, it is hardly a "virtual" copy of bipolar disorder in humans.

> *Diseases such as hypertension, diabetes, and cancer can be more readily studied in animals where organs can be probed after such conditions are created in the animal. Scientists have so far not found any animal models of bipolar disorder.*

Despite our increasing understanding of how medications affect neurotransmitter systems and their receptors, these research limitations have restricted our understanding of how these systems are disordered and thereby lead to and maintain a state of mental illness. Research has revealed some information in this area, however. Studies have discovered increased densities of serotonin receptors in the brains of depressed suicide victims, and correlated low serotonin turnover or function in the brain, with violent suicide (e.g., violent methods such as guns, jumping from high places, or hanging as opposed to overdoses or self-poisoning) and impulsive, sometimes aggressive behavior.

Based on current studies, it is known that most antidepressant medications act to block a transporter site on a nerve ending that takes up the neurotransmitters previously released by this nerve terminal. This is hypothesized to result in a slower breakdown of the neurotransmitters and, therefore, an increased effect on receptors in the space between nerve endings, as well as on receptors on the adjacent nerve cell body. This results in a decrease in the number of receptors on the adjacent nerve cell (called a down regulation), which requires several weeks to occur—about the same length of time required for depression to improve significantly in response to antidepressant medication. This was considered a basic mechanism of the effect of antidepressant medications on clinical depression. In recent years, interest has focused on the "messenger systems" that are activated in the post-synaptic cell by receptors on the cell surface. There are studies suggesting that lithium has the ability to stabilize membranes and perhaps enhance serotonin function by an effect on certain second messenger systems in the cell. There is no clear understanding of the mechanism of divalproex (Depakote) or carbamazepine (Tegretol) in bipolar disorder mood stabilization. It is thought that these medications affect mood stabilization by effects on the neurotransmitter glutamate, but this evidence is limited.

While these studies have yielded few definite conclusions on how neurotransmitters mediate the symptoms of bipolar disorder, they provide direction for the application of newer techniques to get at some of these questions. Researchers have had to devise other methods for getting inside the "black box," the relatively inaccessible human brain, to try to understand the workings of its complex chemical machinery (see Imaging Studies, page 67). As just one measure of its complexity, the brain is composed of at least 40 million functional neurons, each with an average of 5,000 connections with other neurons.

Transduction Systems

One research effort is to find candidate genes that control the formation and metabolism of the neurotransmitters, their receptors, and other complex messenger systems activated by the receptors. The study of the effects of medications such as lithium on these messenger systems is a relatively new and promising direction in research. Focusing on the systems that integrate the effects of neurotransmitters and receptors may circumvent some of the research difficulties outlined above because these systems operate as the final common pathways of the effects of all of the neurotransmitters. They are considered "transduction systems" because they multiply and communicate the sum total of effects of neurotransmitters, while simultaneously affecting genes that may alter the production of both neurotransmitters and receptors.

Neurotrophins and New Cell Production

Scientists have begun to explore an entire area of neurotropic factors now being measured in the brain. Additional studies illustrate clear evidence of neurogenesis (new cell production occurring in the brain). Later you will read of evidence that chronic depressive illness and bipolar disorders, as well as certain anxiety disorders such as PTSD (post-traumatic stress disorder), actually cause a loss of nerve cells in both frontal areas of the brain and the hippocampus (see figure 3.2).

In a paper from Dr. Manji's group, another interesting and possibly optimistic finding is mentioned: "The expression of different genes, including transcription factors, is markedly altered by lithium administration. Chronic lithium treatment also robustly increases the expression of the neuroprotective protein Bcl2, raising the intriguing possibility that some of lithium's effects are mediated through underappreciated neurotrophic (induction of new neuron growth) and neuroprotective effects."[9] This is a revolutionary new understanding of brain function since until recently we have accepted the dictum that new brain cells do not occur, that we simply slowly lose the cells we were born with as we age.

Work like that of Dr. Manji illustrates the effect that certain medications have regarding new cell production. Recent research is also producing evidence that new cell formation (neurogenesis) can be induced in selected areas of the brain of laboratory animals by way of exercise and new learning.

Recent work has taken this step further. Molecular geneticists from Princeton University, under the direction of Dr. J. Z. Tsien, have succeeded in accomplishing a new technique to "knock out" the gene required for the development of an area within the brain that confers non-spatial intelligence on mice. The ability to create a genetic effect that involves only "one" area and function of brain development is an amazing feat! These scientists went further. They placed a group of mice, bred for low intelligence, inside a barren cage and an equal number (also bred for low intelligence) into cages equipped with running wheels, tunnels, and mazes to provide a novel environment. Astonishingly, the "mentally dull" mice inside the enriched environment illustrated the acquisition of abilities and intelligence for which there was no genetic basis.

On close examination, this group of scientists discovered the growth of new nerve endings in the affected areas of the brain tissue of these genetically altered mice. The environmentally enriched group had been provided with the ability to transfer and develop new functions despite their innate lack of such genetic programming.[10]

> Research is producing evidence that new cell formation (neurogenesis) can be induced in selected areas of the brain of laboratory animals by way of exercise and new learning.

The jump from mice to men may be a long one, but it is this very type of "revolutionary" new evidence that raises an important question: Can the biological functioning of the human nervous system be shaped by new learning? If intensive "cognitive therapy" works for mice, it could possibly work for man to help reverse genetic vulnerabilities at the biological level.

Imaging Studies

It appears that our knowledge of the important neurotransmitters, combined with the emerging field of molecular genetics, is allowing us to "leapfrog" some of the barriers to learning about neurotransmitter function in the brain.

The development of brain imaging techniques has allowed researchers to get inside that black box of the human brain without invading the brain itself. This technology makes it possible to pinpoint anatomical differences and detect functional alterations in various areas of the brains of patients with bipolar disorder. Introduced 10 years ago, initial brain imaging efforts focused on defining the differences between bipolar patients and people without the disease. Imaging has now evolved to studying the differences in aspects of brain structure and function between patients with schizophrenia, bipolar disorder, and recurrent depression. This methodology, together with molecular biology and genetic approaches, promises to further advance our knowledge of human brain function.

> It appears that our knowledge of the important neurotransmitters, combined with the emerging field of molecular genetics, is allowing us to "leapfrog" some of the barriers to learning about neurotransmitter function in the brain.

Brain imaging techniques have the advantage of not employing x rays to produce the image and thus avoid the toxicity of excessive doses of radiation. Instead, imaging uses modified radio waves and strong magnetic fields to form images of the atoms and molecules that make up the brain.

Techniques such as magnetic resonance imaging (MRI) "image" brain structures and certain aspects of function, such as blood flow. A related technique, magnetic resonance imaging spectoscopy (MRI-S) allows measurement of certain chemical changes reflecting neuronal function in small areas of the brain. Through this type of imaging, we can measure various chemicals in targeted areas of the brain without interfering with their activity.

Another promising technique, positron emission tomography (PET), can measure metabolic processes in the brain and body. Much can be learned from measuring the rate of metabolism of glucose, a major brain nutrient, in various areas of the brain in distinct disease states such as mania and depression. Specific neurotransmitters are "labeled" with radioisotopes and their function studied in various brain neural circuits.

The PET scans labeled "Depressed Brain" and "Recovered Brain" in the insert show the brain of a patient during depression and after recovery from depression. The colors in the scans correspond to glucose metabolic rates (which indicate activity of the neurons), with the lowest rates associated with the coolest end of the color spectrum (blue) and the highest rates with the warmest (red). If an area that normally reflects higher rates (red, yellow, or green) shows up blue on the scan, it implies that the neurons in that region are impaired in their function. The image made during a depressive episode (left) is dark, mostly blue, whereas the image created after treatment with medication (right) has more green, yellow, and red, showing that the activity of the neurons has normalized.

The second page of the insert shows PET scans of the brain of a drug-free rapid-cycling manic-depressive patient. The images in the top row were made when the patient was depressed. The second row shows the identical planes scanned the next day, when the patient had become manic. The third row shows scans taken 10 days later when the same patient was again depressed. The scans show that the brain is in an abnormal metabolic state (either decreased or increased metabolic function) when the patient is in a depressed or manic state compared with the rates of metabolism measured in the brain during periods of normal function.

These imaging techniques, guided by knowledge gained from studies elucidating the important neurotransmitter systems (despite all the limitations encountered), are leading to rapid advances in our understanding of bipolar disorder and other conditions. At this point, the techniques are purely investigational; they are not developed to a degree that they can be used in clinical treatment. While imaging points to functional and structural abnormalities in illnesses such as bipolar disorder, there is still some variation and inevitable lack of agreement from study to study because of the use of varying techniques and small numbers of patients. The findings are therefore unreliable for diagnosis and treatment decisions.

Valuable findings are emerging from these pioneer advances, and there is great promise for new understanding as these techniques become more powerful. One early finding was that certain left-sided frontal brain damage caused by stroke or trauma may lead to the development of major depression. Post-stroke mania is associated with a right-sided brain injury and either an underlying subcortical loss of cells or a genetic vulnerability to bipolar disorder.

A recent report confirmed previous observations of neuroanatomic deep white matter changes (sometimes called unidentified bright objects, UBOs), as well as subcortical grey matter changes, in primarily young bipolar patients. Both PET and functional-MRI studies have shown decreased metabolism of various areas of the frontal lobes as well as in subcortical structures such as the basal ganglia.

A recent study of cell density in these same brain areas, using tissue taken from individuals dying while in an episode of depression (some with no prior treatment), has shown both reduced neuronal and glial cells (the metabolic support cells for neurons), which corresponds to both PET hypofunction findings and MRI studies revealing signs of atrophy in some patients with these disorders.

> *Recent studies show the brain to be very plastic with evidence of cell atrophy and loss in response to severe prolonged stress and untreated depression. New evidence is emerging that treatment (antidepressants, divalproex, and lithium) may reverse some of these processes.*

Other MRI studies of bipolar patients have revealed atrophy of frontal, temporal, and subcortical areas. Though older patients showed a higher percentage of this trend, the finding appeared in 10 to15 percent of adolescent patients, suggesting an illness-related process. MRI-S allows a measure of changes in certain biochemicals in the living brain. Studies in bipolar patients have revealed decreases of the neurotransmitter glutamate in the anterior cingulate cortex (see figure 3.1) of patients with depression. These findings should be viewed with the awareness that recent studies are showing the brain to be very plastic with evidence of cell atrophy and loss in response to severe prolonged stress and untreated depression. New evidence, reviewed above, is emerging that treatment (antidepressants, divalproex, and lithium) may reverse some of these processes.

Other studies have demonstrated signs of stimulation of neurotrophic and neuroprotective factors in the brains of bipolar patients taking lithium for their disorder.

SUMMARY

Review of the research on the biology of bipolar disorder reveals evident progress in molecular genetics and imaging studies. Additionally, investigations into the effects of medications on key neurotransmitters and messenger systems have significantly increased our knowledge of the brain and the systems affected by bipolar disorder.

Relating findings from one set of methods to another (e.g., effects of medications related to findings on imaging studies), is leading us closer to knowledge that will result in the development of more effective treatments for bipolar disorder and possible earlier diagnosis techniques and prevention strategies. Practical breakthroughs in early diagnosis and treatment will occur unpredictably as further research leads to new paradigms for understanding the biology of bipolar disorder. In the meantime, we must continue research into maximizing the effectiveness of new classes of medications developed to treat bipolar disorder. In the next chapter, we will examine the latest medication strategies and treatment models.

CHAPTER 4

Medication Therapy

THE PAST 35 years have witnessed great progress in the treatment of bipolar disorder and clinical depression. The development of safer, more effective, and easier-to-use medications has brightened the outlook for people who have depressive and manic-depressive conditions. With the increasing volume of research and the continued development of new medications, we see promise of even more effective treatments on the horizon.

Despite the already considerable progress, many unanswered questions and doubts remain about the use of medications in the treatment of clinical depression. Some people find it hard to understand why a medication is necessary to treat what they mistakenly view as a purely psychological disturbance affecting only the mind. In actuality, mental illness results in a wide range of effects on all levels: physical, mental, emotional, and behavioral. Bipolar illness goes to the very center of a person's being, obstructing the ability to enjoy or appreciate life, see beyond oneself, and be productive or creative. Hopelessness and despair are common by-products. Other typical effects include lack of energy and motivation, impaired insight and judgment, and a predisposition to physical illness. Bipolar disorder often extends way beyond the distortion of emotional responses, as it has a profound impact on the body's physiology and the brain's capacity to function.

Not understanding all of this, some people believe that those who experience depression would benefit from learning how to cope more effectively with life's disappointments. "Just deal with it," patients so often hear from others. "Count your blessings" or "confess your sins and turn to God" are other common responses to those suffering from depression. Other people are under the misconception that suffering from depression or mood swings that require medication is a sign of weakness or a "cop-out." Still others believe the person is overlooking a simple panacea. "Try running every day. You'll feel better," some well-meaning friend or relative might say.

Some of these views undoubtedly originate from the stigma associated with a mental disorder, a belief in "true grit," or the concept of "will power." The idea that depression might be the manifestation of some dysfunction of brain mechanisms, and not purely a mind problem that can be overcome by "trying harder," is a difficult concept for skeptics to accept. As a variation on this, some people find a talking treatment (psychotherapy) philosophically easier to embrace than the idea of medication.

> *The idea that depression might be the manifestation of some dysfunction of brain mechanisms, and not purely a mind problem that can be overcome by "trying harder," is a difficult concept for skeptics to accept.*

Unfortunately, the stigma surrounding bipolar disorder is not limited to the general population. It exists in the health-care industry as well, as evidenced by discrimination against paying for the treatment of "mental" disorders as if they are separate and distinct from "medical" disorders. Psychiatric patients have long suffered from drastic cuts in the funding of care that has resulted in denial of coverage for mental illness. Health insurance covers expensive, highly technological procedures such as liver and heart transplants without question. Meanwhile, suicide is the eighth cause of death overall and the third cause of death among people 15 to 24 years old. Many of these deaths could be prevented by access to effective treatment, which is now frequently lacking due to insufficient medical coverage.

The failure of health-care providers to recognize mental illness as a legitimate health problem has reinforced the social stigma, contributed to a rise in mental disorders as they go untreated, and increased the cost to society.

THE UNDERTREATMENT OF BIPOLAR DISORDER AND DEPRESSION

In 1997, National Depressive and Manic-Depressive Association (National DMDA) published *Expert Consensus Treatment Guidelines for Bipolar Disorder: A Guide for Patients and Families*. The report brought to light some damning facts, particularly regarding the long delay between the first onset of symptoms and correct diagnosis and treatment. The report revealed that people with bipolar disorder see approximately three to four doctors and spend more than eight years seeking treatment before they receive a correct diagnosis. The report also pointed to the inability of some primary care providers to make a proper diagnosis because of their limited experience in dealing with psychiatric problems. The attending physician may lack sufficient information on the diagnosis and treatment of depression. In addition, many providers have limited training in managing emotional distress because general practitioners normally deal with physical ailments. This, of course, points to the importance of increased public as well as medical awareness of these disorders.

This report followed a 1996 National DMDA conference to investigate the reasons for the undertreatment of depression. A panel composed of psychiatrists, psychologists, family practitioners, internists, managed care and public health specialists, and members of the community considered six key questions: 1) Is depression undertreated in both the community and the clinic? 2) What is the economic cost to society regarding depression? 3) What have been the

National Depressive and Manic-Depressive Association

Headquartered in Chicago, the National Depressive and Manic-Depressive Association (National DMDA) is the nation's largest patient-run, "illness-specific" organization. It is a major source of support for people with unipolar and bipolar disorders. Since its inception in 1986, members have been working to combat the public stigma surrounding these illnesses. Rather than bow to stigma, members act to obliterate it through education. Public education remains one of the primary purposes of the organization.

efforts in the past to redress undertreatment and how successful have they been? 4) What are the reasons for the gap between our knowledge of the diagnosis and treatment of depression to the actual treatment received in the United States? 5) What can we do to narrow this gap? and 6) What can we do immediately to narrow this gap?

The panel arrived at the following conclusions:

1. Depressive disorders affect 15% of the male population and 24% of females, an increase over the past several generations; the age of onset has also decreased. In a 1980 survey, approximately one-third of the people suffering depression sought treatment. Of those who sought treatment, only about one in ten received adequate help. Unfortunately, the vast majority of patients treated with antidepressants are prescribed an inadequate dose for an insufficient period of time. Although effective psychotherapies exist, few patients receive them or, when they do go for help, the allotted time frame is too short.

2. Depression is one of the ten most costly illnesses in the United States and imposes an enormous burden on society. The many costs and consequences include decreased quality of life for patients and families, high morbidity and mortality, and substantial economic

National DMDA has a grassroots network of 275 chapters and support groups and is managed by an administrative board of directors, the majority of whom are patients themselves. It is also guided by a 65-member Scientific Advisory Board composed of the leading researchers and clinicians in the field of depressive illnesses. Contact DMDA for free educational material, membership information, or to locate a patient-run chapter or support group in your community (see the appendix, "Resources for Information").

losses. A conservative estimate from a recent study calculated the annual national cost of depression at $43 billion. A new cost-benefit analysis estimated that the savings of appropriately treating depression outweighed the direct treatment costs by about $4 billion per year.

3. Educational programs have substantially improved public knowledge and understanding of depression. The D/ART (Depression/Awareness, Recognition, and Treatment) program, sponsored by NIMH (National Institute for Mental Health), provides broadly based outreach to patients, the public, and professionals. NPECCD (National Public Education Campaign on Clinical Depression) is a national, private-sector, nongovernmental program sponsored by the National Mental Health Association and cosponsored by National DMDA, American Psychiatric Association (APA), National Alliance for the Mentally Ill, D/ART, and more than 100 other organizations. Other educational avenues include community

Depression is one of the ten most costly illnesses in the United States and imposes an enormous burden on society. A conservative estimate from a recent study calculated the annual national cost of depression at $43 billion.

programs, public relations efforts, pamphlet distribution for patient information, professional education, and employee assistance programs to benefit workers at their place of employment.

4. The gap between our knowledge of correct treatment of depression and what actually gets implemented can be attributed to patient, provider, and health-care system factors.

Patients: Patients don't recognize the existence of a problem, fail to identify the problem as depression, or underestimate its severity. Some face limited access to treatment or are unwilling to stay with a recommended medical regimen. Many still experience a stigma attached to mental health issues, which, while it is decreasing, remains a reality of our culture and is often reinforced in families.

Providers: Medical schools may fail to provide sufficient education about psychiatric diagnosis, psychopharmacology, or psychotherapy for depression. Other problems include physicians may be inadequately prepared to use the most modern methods; primary care providers may not believe psychiatric disorders are real illnesses; poor insurance coverage; inadequate dosage of antidepressants administered to patients; and some patients' reluctance to see a psychiatrist or other mental health care specialist.

Health-Care System: Some reasons for less than optimal treatment of depression include inadequate insurance reimbursement, lack of qualified specialists, cost-saving plans that discourage treatment and proper monitoring of patients, and insufficient follow-up care.

5. There is a need for additional research and analysis to narrow the gap between diagnosis/treatment determination and actual treatment of depression. The panel designed a slate of questions to help investigate this problem.

6. What can be done immediately to help narrow the gap? Increasing the knowledge of patients and families about treatment options/essential treatment requirements for depression diverts responsibility away from the providers and places it back in the hands of the afflicted. Developing performance standards for behavioral health care can make providers accountable for their standards of treatment. Other proposals included increasing provider knowledge and awareness about new effective treatment and screening for depression; increased collaboration among primary care providers, psychiatrists, and other mental health specialists; and giving more attention to further research, especially as it relates to children, adolescents, and senior citizens.[1]

EFFECTIVENESS OF PSYCHOTHERAPY

Psychotherapies are relatively untested in bipolar disorder. On the other hand, new evidence exists to support the effectiveness of interpersonal and cognitive psychotherapies in unipolar depression of mild to moderate severity. Evidence is mounting that a combination of medication and psychotherapy provides the best results for most patients with depression. Early studies have also shown the ability of family education to improve the outcome of bipolar disorder. In chapter 5, we discuss the benefits of psychotherapy in detail.

> Evidence is mounting that a combination of medication and psychotherapy provides the best results for most patients with depression.

Clearly, psychotherapy ("talk therapy") can be helpful in dealing with issues that otherwise might aggravate bipolar disorder or depression even while a patient is under medication. It is simplistic and counterproductive to view psychotherapy and medication as competing treatments. These modalities are frequently complementary, and each should be utilized when indicated.

The outcome will be poor when an attempt is made to replace one modality with the other, rather than address the aspects of the problem with the appropriate treatment. At this point, the evidence supports the need for mood stabilizers and, possibly, added antidepressants for bipolar disorder. Mood stabilizers, such as lithium or divalproex (Depakote), and olanzepine (Zyprexa), address manic and/or hypomanic (mildly manic) cycles. Antidepressants address breakthrough depression, which is frequently the most common problem in bipolar disorder. The addition of psychotherapy (the appropriate type) depends largely on what other disorders or individual problems need addressing. These may include low self-esteem, excess perfectionism, problems in relationships, poor compliance (with taking prescribed medication), and family problems.

WHEN ARE MEDICATIONS A NECESSARY FORM OF TREATMENT?

During episodes of mania, symptoms of agitation and psychosis may occur. These can result in a state of high energy, with a rush of thoughts and a suspension of self-criticism (or concern about outside criticism, for that matter), which leads to a positive feeling of creativity. Commonly, mania leads to an overestimation of performance since self-criticism is suspended in this mind state. In a minority of cases, the individual is more capable of a real sense of creativity, sometimes resulting in significant accomplishment.

Patients frequently are reluctant to have this state of mind "taken away" by the use of mood-stabilizing medications. Without mood stabilizers, those who feel more creative and generative during a hypomanic episode, but, in fact, are merely oblivious to realistic feedback, may end up suffering from an exercise of poor judgment. For them, it is clear that medication is in their best interest. For the small minority of individuals whose creative achievements were the by-products of hypomania, reluctance to take mood stabilizers is understandable.

Both manic and hypomanic mood swings are frequently followed by episodes of depression, which are usually not prevented by antidepressant medications alone. The question becomes not only what are the consequences of mania, but what is the cost of the depression that is likely to follow? In many cases, the creative period is not worth the suffering from the resulting depression. Nevertheless, this is a decision that must be addressed on an individual basis between the patient and his or her doctor.

There is no question that a role exists in both depression and bipolar disorder for learning new adaptive skills to better cope with life. Learning strategies to increase self-esteem, manage stress, and deal with interpersonal relationships through various types of psychotherapy are often helpful if an individual is in an appropriate state to respond to such interventions; the person must be functioning well enough to derive benefit from therapy.

People with mood swings associated both with the milder and the more severe forms of bipolar disorder require the appropriate medication to control their imbalance. There is also some evidence that more severe depressions, characterized by more severe symptoms, prolonged duration, greater impairment of function, and increased suicidal risk respond more reliably and positively to medications.

A large and growing body of information confirms the theory (which the authors adhere to) that more severe forms of clinical depression and bipolar disorder are associated with biochemical brain changes. These changes in brain chemistry are more likely to develop in individuals with a family history of clinical depression and bipolar disorder, just as diabetes and high blood pressure tend to occur in families with a history of those disorders. Newer medical imaging

> Both manic and hypomanic mood swings are frequently followed by episodes of depression, which are usually not prevented by antidepressant medications alone. The question becomes not only what are the consequences of mania, but what is the cost of the depression that is likely to follow?

techniques can demonstrate a change of the metabolism in specific areas of the brain commonly associated with depression (see color insert photos). Most of these brain changes will return to normal after successful treatment.

WHEN THE USE OF MEDICATION IS INDICATED

Patients with mood swings of mania or hypomania require treatment with mood-stabilizing medications (e.g., lithium, divalproex, and possibly other medications that will be discussed later). Untreated mood swings usually become more frequent and more severe rather than showing improvement over time.

Periods of depression frequently develop following periods of mania or hypomania. In some instances, milder symptoms will improve with mood stabilizers alone, sometimes results will be seen after increasing the dosage, or the addition of lithium may be indicated if not previously prescribed. It is common for depression to become chronic, or to continually recur and become a major obstacle for patients with both bipolar I and bipolar II disorders. Depression can produce disability, ruined careers, marital problems, a life without happiness, or even suicide.

In these more severe forms of depression, antidepressant medications are indicated despite an increased risk of inducing manic or hypomanic cycles. The risk of this problem is much less if mood-stabilizing medications are being used in adequate doses prior to the use of antidepressant medications. In the case of severely worsening symptoms or prolonged depression, the risk of a mood cycle is outweighed by the pain, damage, and suicidal risk of severe depression. If a person in this situation mentions suicide, or wishes to die, it is imperative that lethal weapons or substances are removed and a physician, preferably a psychiatrist, is contacted. The patient should not be left alone until properly evaluated.

CHOOSING AND EVALUATING MEDICATIONS

For many years, doctors treating depression and manic-depression had few options to choose from. In the 1980s and 1990s, however, the Food and Drug Administration (FDA) approved several new mood-stabilizing and antidepressant drugs including serotonin reuptake inhibitors, an anticonvulsant, and an atypical antipsychotic medication for depression and bipolar disorder. These newer drugs are as effective as the older medications, while being safer and better tolerated.

The goal of mood-stabilizing medication (including lithium, the anticonvulsant, divalproex, and the atypical antipsychotic, olanzepine) is the moderation or prevention of mood cycles, ideally for both mania (or hypomania) and depression. By controlling mania, these medications also limit the damage resulting from the impaired judgment that accompanies mania. While there have long been studies supporting the use of lithium, during the 1980s, anticonvulsants such as carbamazepine (Tegretol), and later divalproex (Depakote), were found helpful in mood stabilization. Depakote was later approved for use in acute bipolar disorder. More recently, an atypical antipsychotic medication, olanzepine (Zyprexa), has been approved for the treatment of acute mania in bipolar disorder. We are just beginning to learn how mood stabilizers work.

Since the early 1970s anticonvulsant drugs have shown considerable therapeutic promise in the treatment of manic episodes even before being approved by the FDA. Antidepressant medications decrease or eliminate "target symptoms" of clinical depression both in unipolar and bipolar disorder. However, the severity and debilitating effects of the depressive target symptoms vary from patient to patient. One patient may have no energy or motivation, sleep all day, and be prone to weight gain. Another patient may appear anxious and sleepless, with poor concentration and little to no appetite.

In each of these cases, a medication strategy would be designed to fit the patient's needs in minimizing target symptoms. The most important principle to keep in mind in choosing medication is a patient's individual response. While one person with bipolar disorder or depression may experience a vast improvement with medication X, another patient with similar symptoms may not benefit at all or suffer too many unwanted side effects. This patient might respond better to medication Y.

Sometimes several different medication trials, or a combination of medications, may be necessary to achieve sufficient improvement. The patient's prior experience with medication is a good predictor of what drugs to try or to avoid. A personal record of treatment, including medication and dosages used, the length of time taken, and any positive or negative experiences, can be a valuable tool for the doctor in determining a medication strategy.

> With a successful course of medication, the symptoms of depression should decrease, if not totally disappear. This should occur within 2 to 8 weeks, but a full response sometimes takes 12 to 16 weeks.

With a successful course of medication, the symptoms of depression should decrease, if not totally disappear. This should occur within 2 to 8 weeks, but a full response sometimes takes 12 to 16 weeks. Some patients may require more than one course of treatment (or medication trial) to attain a good result. For others, improvement may occur even though troubles, such as a problematic relationship or unsuccessful living style, remain. Psychotherapy may be necessary in these cases since medications benefit a patient by reducing or removing the symptoms of depression, not by changing negative life situations. As depressed patients improve, their ability to cope with life's adversities also improves.

It is important for patients to continue antidepressant medications long after their depressive symptoms have disappeared in order to avoid a relapse or recurrence. If medication is stopped prematurely, or without a gradual tapering of the dose, a relapse will occur. In the case of bipolar patients, antidepressants are often gradually discontinued after a stable response is obtained, while mood stabilizers are continued indefinitely.

Generally, the first one to three months is considered necessary to establish acute response to treatment, with a subsequent six months on a stable effective dose of medication as a continuation phase to ensure stabilization and prevent a relapse. Depending on the duration of the depressive episode, and the number and severity of prior episodes, a doctor may recommend maintenance treatment for one to several years, and sometimes indefinitely, since depression is often a recurring condition. We have evidence from a number of studies that symptom relapse rates are high if medications are not continued long enough. In the case of patients with bipolar disorder who take mood stabilizers, antidepressants may be tapered and discontinued somewhat earlier.

> It is important for patients to continue antidepressant medications long after their depressive symptoms have disappeared in order to avoid a relapse or recurrence. If medication is stopped prematurely, or without a gradual tapering of the dose, a relapse will occur.

Just as patients with diabetes or high blood pressure must remain on their medication, those with bipolar disorder, who suffer recurrent depression and chronic depression, need long-term medication, which can prevent most, or all, of the recurrences that characterize the illness. Once symptomatic and diagnosed, bipolar disorder is likely to be recurrent for a lifetime if left untreated.

TYPES OF MEDICATION

Most clinicians go through a sequence of trial and error before deciding on the best course of treatment for a patient with bipolar disorder. The nature and severity of the illness will determine the type of drug therapy. Options include antidepressants, mood stabilizers, anticonvulsants, and newer "antipsychotic" medications. Whatever drug or combination of drugs is indicated, the patient must be monitored for side effects.

How Do Psychiatric Drugs Work?

When you take a pill for some physical ailment, you can usually see or feel the results of the medication, often within a reasonable amount of time. An aspirin will make your headache go away, and an antibiotic will cure your infection. But what do psychiatric drugs do?

Most psychiatric medications act in the brain to either increase or decrease the effects of various neurotransmitters (which send chemical messages from nerve cell to nerve cell). This process attempts to normalize brain function.

Mood Stabilizers and Anticonvulsant Medication

The FDA has approved three primary medications for the treatment of bipolar disorder: lithium, divalproex (Depakote), and olanzepine (Zyprexa). As discussed previously, lithium is a mood stabilizer; Depakote is an anticonvulsant, as is carbamazepine. The latter is not FDA-approved for treatment of bipolar disorder but is sometimes used "off label." (Doctors can prescribe medications that have been approved for other illnesses.)

Olanzepine, the most recently approved medication, is classified as an atypical neuroleptic (antipsychotic). New medications that are currently being studied to establish their effectiveness are also in use.

Lithium: Lithium, a natural element, was the first medication on the market for the treatment of manic-depression. Approved by the FDA in the 1970s for bipolar disorder, lithium is sold under numerous brand names: Lithobid, Lithonate, Lithotabs, Cibalith-S, Eska-lith, and Eskalith-CR. A mood stabilizer, lithium is used to treat the manic phase of bipolar disorder and prevent a recurrence of manic and/or depressive episodes. Once the mania subsides, lithium is administered on a maintenance basis.

Scientists have not yet determined the specifics of how lithium works, but it is believed that lithium corrects chemical imbalances that occur in certain brain cells. The drug can be effective when used alone, or in combination with other medications. For example, medicines that had been initially approved for the prevention of temporal lobe epilepsy (carbamazepine and divalproex) are now administered in combination with lithium to treat bipolar disorder. Lithium is also being used to augment the effects of antidepressant medication when the response is less than optimal.

Divalproex sodium (Depakote): Divalproex sodium was first developed for the treatment of epilepsy. Since the FDA approved its use for acute mania in 1995, doctors and patients have relied on it for both acute and long-term treatment.

Although as an anticonvulsant its mechanism of action is different from that of lithium, divalproex sodium has the same effect and may benefit patients who do not respond well to either lithium or carbamazepine. Patients may also tolerate this drug better than they do either of the other ones. Additionally, divalproex sodium works very effectively during manic episodes of bipolar disorder and acts to reduce the severity of future mood swings.

Carbamazepine (Atretol and Tegretol): Another anticonvulsant, carbamazepine, is used as an alternative to lithium and divalproex sodium. Originally marketed for seizure disorders such as epilepsy, carbamazepine has been used more recently for patients with bipolar disorder. It specifically helps to keep the manic phase of bipolar disorder under control, and it has been very effective (alone or in combination with lithium) in the treatment of patients with rapid-cycling bipolar disorder. Additionally, patients who first experience a depressive episode before an attack of mania may benefit from taking carbamazepine, either alone or combined with lithium.

New medications: Newer anticonvulsants, which may have mood-stabilizing effects and are currently being tested, include gabapentin (Neurontin), camotrigine (Lamictal), and topirimate (Topomax).

Topomax, the third anticonvulsant now being tested, is of particular interest because of its association with weight loss. Weight gain is a side effect associated with lithium and Depakote.

Olanzepine (Zyprexa) was recently approved for the treatment of bipolar disorder. This represents a promising new class of agents ("mood normalizers") that not only treat psychosis but help with mania, depression, agitation, and anxiety—often exhibited in bipolar patients. Another new and promising agent, resperidone (Resperidal) is being further studied. Other similar drugs, such as ziprasidone (Zeldox), may prove helpful and effective for future use in bipolar disorder.

Side Effects of Lithium and Other Mood Stabilizers

The following are steps you can take to reduce the side effects of lithium, other mood stabilizers, and anticonvulsants and use these drugs more safely:

Have blood tests. Your doctor should test your blood regularly if you are taking lithium. Testing is necessary more often in the initial stages of taking the medication. Once your doctor has determined the appropriate dosage and your blood levels of lithium have stabilized, a blood test every six months to one year is advisable. This will rule out rare effects on the kidney or on the thyroid.

Elderly individuals are typically more sensitive to lithium and, therefore, may require a lower dosage than younger adults. Lithium can be dangerous for people on low-sodium diets or those who have lost sodium through severe vomiting or diarrhea, and for people who have kidney disease. This is because lithium tends to replace lost sodium in the body, leading to increasing blood levels that can be toxic. Lithium toxicity presents with nausea, vomiting, impaired coordination of movements or gait, and mental confusion as well as kidney damage. Lithium toxicity is a medical emergency.

Adjust medication dosage. Even when lithium blood levels are in the correct range, side effects can, and do, occur, although this varies widely from patient to patient. Some patients may notice a fine tremor of their hands. This symptom may be more prominent with fine movements or under social performance stress, as in holding and drinking from a cup in a group of people. The tremor is not a sign of serious toxicity, but it is bothersome socially. Sometimes a small decrease in the lithium dose helps; in other cases, switching to another medication is an answer.

Take medication at night. When you are on lithium, you may notice a tendency to urinate more frequently than usual. You also may experience increased thirst. This is usually a benign, if somewhat inconvenient, side effect. It may help to take your lithium in the evening, but only if your doctor thinks it's safe for you to do so.

Put things in perspective. Lithium can worsen acne and make your hair thin and brittle. Some people feel that they experience mental dulling or less creativity on lithium, but this is rare. It is wise to view the side effects of lithium in the context of its effectiveness in helping to prevent the social and career consequences of mania and the suffering and disability of depression and mood swings that can dominate your life.

Don't suddenly stop taking lithium. Recent evidence has accumulated in the European literature suggesting that lithium maintenance actually lowers the risk of suicide in bipolar and perhaps unipolar patients as well. But research also shows that a sudden discontinuation of lithium results in a higher likelihood of rapid mood swings into mania and may increase suicide risk.[2]

Watch for other side effects. Depakote is usually well tolerated, but it can cause nausea. Certain antacids (Pepcid) may keep this symptom in check. Drowsiness can occur if the blood level of Depakote is too high. This is easily remedied, however, by adjusting the dosage. A tremor is also a possibility, but a slight lowering of the dosage frequently regulates this, too.

Alert doctor to reaction. It is very important to inform both the doctor who prescribed your medication and your family doctor of any symptoms you experience. You should do so even if you don't think there's a connection between the medication and the symptom. By way of illustration, a rare hypersensitivity to divalproex can cause pancreatitis, a serious condition that usually presents with abdominal pain and distress. Patients don't typically associate accompanying abdominal pain with the medication, but tend to attribute the pain to flu symptoms. They also tend to consult their primary care physician, rather than their psychiatrist who would be aware of rare side effects.

To minimize pharmaceutical side effects, check with your doctor about periodic laboratory testing.

Don't drink and medicate! You should either avoid drinking or be very careful when drinking alcohol if you are taking Depakote or Tegretol because they can increase the sedating effects of alcohol.

When taking Tegretol. Although it happens rarely, Tegretol can cause a drop in white blood cells, so periodic laboratory tests should be taken, especially if you are getting frequent infections, colds, or flu. The body is very sensitive to too much Tegretol. If the blood level is too high, uncoordination and even double vision can result. This is most likely to happen in the initial stages of taking the medication or after a dosage increase. **Safety alert:** If serious skin rashes, blotchiness, and itchiness occur, contact your doctor and stop taking Tegretol immediately. Be aware of possible adverse drug interactions (such as with the antibiotic erythromycin).

Don't take drugs during pregnancy. For women of childbearing age, be aware that lithium can cause an increased risk of congenital heart defects, particularly in the first trimester of pregnancy. Depakote and Tegretol, as well as other anticonvulsants, can lead to serious defects of a baby's nervous system. Since 65 percent of all pregnancies are unanticipated, this subject should be carefully discussed with your doctor.

Antidepressant Medications

The occurrence and severity of side effects from antidepressant medications are difficult to predict in the individual patient. When the physician knows the pharmacologic effects of the medication used, it is possible to estimate which side effects are more likely to occur.

A physician has numerous options in treating a patient who is suffering from depression. More than 20 antidepressant medications are now on the market. Some of these, such as SSRIs (selective serotonin-reuptake inhibitors) and the newer dual-action medications, are safer in terms of overdose toxicity or in having no effect on a diseased heart, as compared with the older TCAs (tricyclic antidepressants). In most patients, the newer medications produce fewer side effects than the older ones.

Before the advent of fluoxetine (Prozac), psychiatrists relied on two classes of antidepressants: TCAs and MAOIs (monoamine oxidase inhibitors). All of these medications are thought to work by increasing the availability of neurotransmitters. The older drugs produced more unpleasant side effects because they affected several different neurotransmitters and were more toxic when overdosed.

Most of the newer antidepressant medications act to increase neurotransmitter activity of the brain. One of the most studied neurotransmitters associated with mood disorders, serotonin is in a class of chemicals called monoamines. Other antidepressant medications have effects on other monoamine neurotransmitters, such as norepinephrine. Since patients with similar symptoms may respond differently with one medication or another, medications that have their therapeutic effect through different chemical mechanisms provide doctors with a wide range of treatment options.

Prozac, approved by the FDA in 1987, was widely accepted because it has fewer side effects than the TCAs and MAOIs. Prozac was the first of the SSRIs. The function of the SSRI is to block only the reabsorption of serotonin and no other neurotransmitters. A second generation of SSRIs (Zoloft and Paxil) followed Prozac.

After serotonin exerts its effect in the brain, enzymes break down the neurotransmitter, which is then flushed out of the body or reabsorbed by the transmitting nerve cells and stored for future use. The latter process is called "reuptake." If the brain is producing an insufficient number of circulating neurotransmitters, and if they are in insufficient concentration to connect with their receptors, or the receptors are in some way unresponsive, it is hypothesized that patients are then vulnerable to depression.[3]

SSRI medications block the reuptake of serotonin, resulting in an increase of serotonin in the synapse. Different SSRI medications, e.g., Serzone and Remeron, have the capacity to block certain serotonin receptors, which may have a tendency to reduce anxiety. Research in neuroscience is identifying other important neurotransmitters and factors affected by newer medications.

As more is known about the neurochemistry of the brain and its alterations in a depressed patient, the capacity to "design" more effective medications with fewer side effects improves. While different medications have different likely effects and side effects, an individual's response to treatment is not predictable. This is because different individuals may respond dissimilarly to the same medication. Sometimes, when it is difficult to attain a good response to treatment, adding a medication (augmenting) or combining certain medications may be helpful.

> As more is known about the neurochemistry of the brain and its alterations in a depressed patient, the capacity to "design" more effective medications with fewer side effects improves.

While some primary care physicians have the training and experience to diagnose depression and prescribe antidepressant medications, others do not. If depressive symptoms persist or are either undiagnosed or unresponsive to two courses of medication, or if suicidal thoughts are present, ask for a referral or contact a psychiatrist. The skillful use of mood stabilizers or antidepressant medications in the treatment of depression can reclaim, even save, a life.

Side Effects of Antidepressants

It must be understood that *all effective medications can have side effects*. These may vary widely in severity from medication to medication and patient to patient. The occurrence of side effects depends on dosage and individual sensitivity. Although most side effects are merely inconvenient or interfere slightly with the quality of one's life, some rare, although medically significant, side effects can occur. Obviously, the benefits of the medication should exceed the difficulties.

A list of possible side effects can be frightening or intimidating to anyone, but especially to a patient who is experiencing distress, anxiety, or hopelessness associated with depression. However, side effects can usually be managed merely by changing medication doses or switching from one medication to another. It is also important to realize that many people will have slight-to-no significant side effects.

It is sometimes difficult to separate side effects from the symptoms of the depression. It is clear that side effects are a factor if symptoms only occur after the initiation or a dose increase of the medication. Side effects usually occur early in the treatment; they rarely begin after weeks of treatment without side effects. When medication therapy is actively reported to and managed by your doctor, the side effects do not interfere with the medical benefits.

Many of the available newer antidepressants are likely to produce only one or two side effects. Most of the side effects of newer medications decrease over a period of one to two weeks. Dosage adjustments may also minimize side effects. Antidepressant medications are not habit forming, and sometimes they are required to be taken for months or years to prevent a relapse. If you decide to stop taking them, do so gradually, and only after consulting with your doctor.

Figure 4.1 summarizes patient reports of side effects from medication in a recent Internet survey of 1,370 people (of which 46 percent were diagnosed with bipolar disorder) who reported on the treatment of their depressive symptoms. Results of the survey, which was conducted by the National DMDA,[1] show that drowsiness and sedation

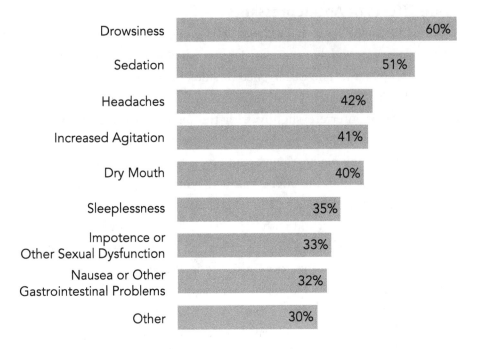

Figure 4.1—*Side Effects Experienced by Depressed Patients While Taking Medication*
(Source: 1999 National Depressive and Manic-Depressive Association online survey.)

are the most commonly reported side effects. Many of these side effects can be managed, or decreased, by reporting them and working with your doctor. None represent a serious medical threat (although you should not drive a car or operate heavy machinery if you experience drowsiness or sedation).

This survey demonstrates that medications require careful management by a physician. It also indicates the need for the development of improved medications with fewer side effects and greater effectiveness.

Alternative Medicines

Since alternative medicine is rapidly becoming popular, let's take a moment to discuss this form of treatment. For our purposes, we will discuss only one herbal and one nutritive supplement.

St. John's wort: The herb St. John's wort (*Hypericum perforatum*) is widely used in Europe to treat mild-to-moderate depression. It is available over the counter in the United States. The FDA does not regulate the purity and potency of St. John's wort products because it is not considered a drug. Although Duke University Medical Center is currently conducting controlled research on St. John's Wort, its effectiveness in treating depression and preventing suicide has not been established.

Andrew Neirenberg, M.D., recently reported two cases of mania resulting in patients who were taking St. John's wort for depression. Any conventional antidepressant medication can precipitate mania in an unrecognized bipolar patient or a bipolar patient who is not mood stabilized. Substances that have positive effects can also have side effects, whether "natural" or designed and manufactured. All of our early medications (e.g., aspirin, digitalis, reserpine—used to treat high blood pressure) were discovered initially in plants.

To learn more about St. John's wort, see Dr. Steven Bratman's book, *Beat Depression with St. John's Wort*.[4]

The Omega Plan: Early positive findings in medical research include the use of omega-3 fatty acids in the treatment of bipolar disorder. It has been reported as a breakthrough dietary plan that replaces harmful fats with beneficial ones. The plan derived from the theory that people who consume a lot of fish (which is high in omega-3 fatty acids that cannot be manufactured in our bodies), as evidenced in Japan, Taiwan, and Hong Kong, have a low rate of depression. But, although we have seen some early results with this new approach that support its effectiveness, it needs further confirmation.

In 1999, Dr. Andrew Stoll, of McLean Hospital and Harvard Medical School, began to study the use of omega-3 fatty acids to treat bipolar disorder. He and his colleagues recruited 30 bipolar outpatients into a double-blind placebo-controlled study over a four-month period. All of these patients had experienced manic or hypomanic episodes within the prior year, and none had responded favorably to lithium or Depakote. The outcome of Stoll's research determined that

> The use of omega-3 fatty acids in the treatment of bipolar disorder is an early positive finding in medical research.

patients on omega-3 fatty acids had a significantly longer period of remission than those in the placebo group. Fifty percent of the patients who had taken placebos relapsed within two months, while none of the 15 patients receiving 6 to 8 grams per day of omega-3 fatty acids relapsed.[5]

The Omega Plan has not been fully tested as an effective measure in treating bipolar disorder. Until further scientific research has been completed, we cannot support the Omega Plan as a substitute for antidepressant drugs. Two months is a short time to test the effect of treatment in bipolar disorder. Dr. Stoll is more completely testing the effects of high dose omega-3 fatty acids.

OUT OF THE CUCKOO'S NEST: ELECTROCONVULSIVE THERAPY TODAY

Electroconvulsive therapy (ECT) was widely used in the 1940s and 1950s and remains the most effective and rapid treatment for severe depression. Although it is vastly safer and more humane today than it was in the past, it is still a controversial and seldom employed therapy.

It is not known exactly how ECT helps both severe and unresponsive bipolar disorder and depression. There is evidence to suggest ECT works by causing a seizure, a state in which most of the brain's systems are stimulated, thereby increasing brain neurotransmitter production. When successful (80 to 90 percent of the time), the effects of this treatment can last several months, although relapse is as high as 50 percent in one year without appropriate maintenance medication. There are side effects with ECT, notably, short-term memory loss, which in most cases gradually disappears.

The attending physician administers a short-acting barbiturate, such as sodium Pentothal (an anesthesia), and a muscle relaxer to the patient. A brief electrical pulse is then given, which causes a brain seizure. Within seconds, the patient's body convulses, appearing to twitch, but without major spasms because of the muscle relaxant. An anesthesiologist usually administers oxygen, and the patient is carefully monitored throughout the procedure.

ECT is used for the most serious forms of psychotic depression in which the depression is severe, often accompanied by suicide risk, and when the patient has not benefited from adequate courses of medication. For these patients, ECT may be a lifesaving treatment. ECT is frequently used in elderly patients who are frail and unable to tolerate or benefit from antidepressant medications. It is unquestionably safer than portrayed in such Hollywood movies as *One Flew Over the Cuckoo's Nest*. The film actually portrayed the most primitive use of ECT as it occurred in the 1940s, before the procedure was developed to its current state and before any other medications were available.

HOW TO AVOID HOSPITALIZATION

When required, hospitalization does not usually continue for longer than one to two weeks. Hospitalization is used as a last resort to protect someone's life or to treat a patient who has not benefited from conventional treatment. Only if a life or a person's future is at risk should admission be forced on a patient. The determination as to the degree of suicide risk is very difficult, and the decision should be made by a qualified medical health professional. Also, hospitalization is required for those individuals who have medical complications that make drug monitoring difficult or impossible. Hospitalization is also a useful course for those patients who have drug or alcohol dependency, in addition to bipolar disorder or clinical depression.

> Hospitalization is used as a last resort to protect someone's life or to treat a patient who has not benefited from conventional treatment. Only if a life or a person's future is at risk should admission be forced on a patient.

Early intervention and treatment of bipolar disorder can help reduce the likelihood of the need for hospitalization. It is important to give serious consideration to slowing down the process so each patient has an opportunity to feel empowered. Hospitalization is appropriate to prevent an imminent suicide or violent act, as well as to treat patients who may be unable to be treated without protective custody. Hospitalization cannot be forced on a patient unless it can be determined that the patient is suicidal, at risk to commit some violent act, or is rendered incapable of physically caring for him- or herself.

TALKING WITH YOUR DOCTOR

It is very important that you have a trusting relationship with your doctor and feel confidence in his or her knowledge, skill, and interest in helping you. On your part, you must convey the information your doctor needs to help you. Always tell your doctor about all medications, "natural" treatments, and other substances you are taking since these substances could interact with medications that are prescribed. A complete medical history including medication reactions, allergies, and prior experiences with medication is important. A skilled and interested doctor will likely address many of the issues contained in the following questions. If he or she doesn't, you may want to ask about these issues so that you are comfortable with and have confidence in your doctor and your course of treatment. Consider the following questions:

What is my medication dosage, and how should I increase it if this is to be done before my next visit? (It is a good idea to write down this information, especially if it is complicated.)

What side effects might I expect, and what should I do if I experience a side effect?

Will mood stabilizers or antidepressants reduce or change either my mental performance or my judgment?

How can I reach the doctor if I experience any severe side effect or worsening of my condition? (Before you leave the appointment, be sure you have an emergency phone number for reaching your doctor.)

When should I expect some improvement, and what type of improvement should I expect?

Are there any hazards associated with taking this treatment and how can I recognize them?

How long will it be necessary to take the medicine?

If the medication needs to be stopped for any reason, how should this be done?

How often will I need to come for an appointment, and how long should the appointment be?

Is any type of psychotherapy recommended as part of the treatment?

Are there activities or other things I can do to improve my response to treatment?

Are there activities I should avoid in order to increase my likelihood of improvement?

If this medication isn't helpful, are there other alternatives for treatment? If so, what are they?

If someone asks me why I need medication, or raises concerns about possible dangers of taking medication, how should I respond?

Voice any concerns you have about taking the recommended medication that you have not talked about.

INTERNET SURVEY RESULTS

The first Internet survey conducted by the National Depressive and Manic-Depressive Association (National DMDA) became available just as this book was going to press.[2] A total of 1,370 people participated in the survey, all of whom had reported symptoms of depression.

We have stressed that currently available treatment can help the vast majority of patients who seek help and are in compliance with their doctor's instructions. Nevertheless, treatment options need to be further expanded and improved. More research can provide additional and more effective medications and psychotherapies.

Of the total participants surveyed, 46 percent were diagnosed with bipolar disorder. Out of this group, 87 percent reported that they had received treatment during the past five years.

As illustrated in table 1, 93 percent of those surveyed experienced depression nearly every day, and for the better portion of the day. Also noted in the survey are loss of interest or pleasure in usual activities, fatigue, and loss of energy.

Some 28 to 35 percent experienced no change of depressed mood or capacity for enjoyment, and 40 percent reported no change regarding fatigue or loss of energy. These results suggest the need for the development of even more effective medications to reduce depressive symptoms, especially fatigue and low energy.

Participants who responded to being "very satisfied" or "somewhat satisfied" with their treatment comprised 61 percent of the sample, while 28 percent reported dissatisfaction (see figure 4.2).

Of those people who followed a course of antidepressant treatment, only 25 percent were still taking the original prescription while

Table 1. Symptoms Before and After Treatment

Symptoms	Before Treatment	After Treatment
Depressed (sad or gloomy) mood most of the day, nearly every day	93%	28%
Loss of interest or pleasure in usual activities most of the day, nearly every day	93%	35%
Fatigue or loss of energy	96%	40%

(Source: Adapted from the 1999 National Depressive and Manic-Depressive online survey.)

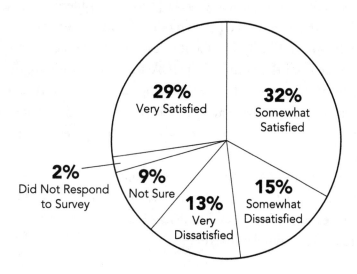

Figure 4.2—*Satisfaction/Dissatisfaction with Treatment*
(Source: 1999 National Depressive and Manic-Depressive Association online Survey.)

75 percent admitted to having discontinued at least one of their pre-scribed medications. Simultaneously, 69 percent said they were con-tinuing to medicate on a regular basis, and as ordered. This number of patients, along with the high percentage who had tried and stopped medication, suggests that many did not benefit from their initial course of treatment and needed to try something different.

Desire for some future medication that does not cause drowsiness, sedation, headaches, tension, or other similar side effects was con-veyed by 80 percent of the participants. Of those patients who had considered not taking antidepressant medication, 23 percent feared that antidepressants would "change their personality." Some with chronic depression felt their personality improved with treatment. Another 18 percent of participants were concerned about the poten-tial for the medication to become habit-forming. To date, we have no substantiating evidence to support that concern. What has been ascertained is the importance of continuing medication to prevent recurring depression.

The survey also confirmed that 35 percent considered not taking antidepressants, these people believing they could manage their symptoms on their own. Finally, 8 percent refused medication entirely.

It is clear from the National DMDA study that while more than 60 percent of those treated reported being helped and were satisfied with treatment, a significant number received no benefit, or only partial benefit, and had core symptoms of the illness remaining after treatment.

These new findings underscore the hope that help can be obtained from proper treatment. But, they also indicate the need for additional research and the development of more effective treatments for depression and bipolar disorder.

SUMMARY

A great deal of progress has been made in the treatment of bipolar disorder and depression, especially with the development of new medications. These treatments are not perfect. Often, either because a medication is not helpful to an individual patient or produces intolerable side effects, more than one trial of medication is necessary. In some cases, it may take a combination of several medications to achieve the desired improvement.

We do not know why one patient responds completely to one mood stabilizer or antidepressant and another patient with similar symptoms has difficulty getting a good response from medication. This is true not only of psychiatric conditions, but with all medical illnesses as well. Patients with ulcers, high blood pressure, arthritis, diabetes, and convulsions (epilepsy) show the same varied patterns of response. This is what makes medicine as much an art as a science.

The expert practitioner must keep up with the latest information on the use of medications and help each individual patient get the best possible response. Finding the right medication may take several trials, for there is limited data to predict response to a given drug in an individual patient. If a response is not forthcoming, it is worth getting a second opinion or an expert consultation. Never give up! Some rare individuals finally find the medication that works after failing to benefit from 10 to 15 treatment trials. The hope is, of course, that you or your loved one will respond well to a first treatment. Keep in mind, however, that sometimes you need to stay with treatment for a longer period and try different methods in order to obtain a good result.

CHAPTER 5

Psychotherapy

THE MOST COMPREHENSIVE and advantageous treatment of bipolar illness should involve medication treatment combined with psychotherapy. While bipolar illness is a medical disorder, it is expressed through one's thoughts, mood, social interaction, physical well-being, behavior, and sense of self. Medication treatment can address the severity of the illness, but those living with bipolar illness need the skills and awareness to both make sense of their illness and to develop proactive and reactive approaches to help minimize the impact of the illness.

Psychotherapy offers those with bipolar illness increased understanding of their illness and an ability to distinguish between the effects of the illness and issues related to normal living. Treatment that is based on an open and trusting therapeutic relationship can help an individual with bipolar illness distinguish between the debilitating aspect of severe depression and natural experiences of sadness and depression. Similarly, psychotherapy offers an understanding of the differences between healthy optimism and the boundless unrealistic optimism associated with severe mania. Psychotherapy also involves an exploration of patterns—in one's thoughts, moods, and behavior. Through such exploration, patients can learn to recognize how daily life events affect them. Similarly, they can learn skills to cope with life's challenges better.

Another function of psychotherapy is to help patients understand the meaning they assign to their illness and how that influences their response to it. For example, while one patient steadfastly complies with medication and views her illness as a part of her life challenge, another so completely embraces his illness, that his self-identity is embedded in "being" bipolar. Psychotherapy can be helpful in exploring issues that are unique to one's personality, such as those related to dependency, free will, optimism, and self-esteem. Psychotherapy can play a tremendous role by helping to influence how a patient responds to living with bipolar illness.

> Psychotherapy offers an understanding of the differences between healthy optimism and the boundless unrealistic optimism associated with severe mania.

Another major challenge that psychotherapy can address is medication compliance. An empathic therapeutic relationship can help people who live with bipolar illness make sense of and manage the many emotions, motivations, and attitudes that influence whether or not they adhere to the recommended medication treatment. In this context, a patient can explore the full range of emotions that accompany the experience of living with bipolar illness.

A psychotherapeutic session offers patients a haven. It is an intimate setting that encourages them to acknowledge their anger and fear. It also enables them to release any competing motivations that play against each other when balancing the pros and cons of medication. Psychotherapy can help the patient recognize and make use of "self-talk": "I want to feel better, but I don't want to give up my energy; I want to feel better, but I don't want to feel dependent on medication to do so; I want to feel better, but I will lose my creativity; I want to feel better, but I don't want to give up that wonderful feeling of being totally unselfconscious when I am manic." Patient and therapist can discuss these subjective experiences so the patient can fully understand and take responsibility for his or her choices in coping with bipolar illness.

For psychotherapy to be effective for individuals with bipolar illness, it must foster increased self-awareness. It is most advantageous when it also helps a patient discover specific skills for problem solving and for coping with the complexity of life's everyday challenges. One form of therapy that addresses these concerns is cognitive behavioral therapy. We should emphasize that this form of psychotherapy is most effective in dealing with depression. Specifically, individuals who exhibit stable moods, mild, moderate, or somewhat severe depression are helped the most. In contrast, those with severe depression or mania lack the capacity for structured and objective self-reflection essential for such therapy. For them, stabilization by medication is a prerequisite for psychotherapy. Finally, those experiencing low levels of mania are minimally motivated to seek treatment. So, it is during depression or periods of greater stability that those with bipolar illness may achieve the best results from this powerful form of treatment.

COGNITIVE BEHAVIOR THERAPY

"I can't do anything right. My life is a complete waste. I am nothing. I am totally inadequate. Nothing is going to change. I might as well give up!"

These are some of the paralyzing thoughts that pervasively dominate one's awareness during severe depression. As viewed by cognitive behavior therapists, it is the intense and compelling nature of such thoughts that deeply influences one's mood and, ultimately, one's behavior and physical well-being. The intensity and pervasiveness of these thoughts and the emotions they arouse leave little room for objective reasoning. These thoughts and the type of thinking that leads to them are the focus of "cognitive restructuring," one form of cognitive behavior therapy. In a collaborative effort, therapist and client work together to identify these thoughts and evaluate, challenge, and, ultimately, replace them with thoughts that are based on more objective reflection.

Two other forms of cognitive behavior therapy are coping skills therapy and problem solving therapy. Coping skills therapy focuses on specific behaviors while problem solving therapy helps individuals develop adaptive means for dealing with everyday life. Some of the cognitive behavioral approaches may fall in more than one category. Comprehensive cognitive behavior therapy draws on each of these approaches in the treatment for those living with bipolar illness.

COGNITIVE RESTRUCTURING

"You feel the way you think," says David Burns, a researcher and author in the area of depression.[1] Hormone problems, chemical imbalance, or other physiological changes can trigger some forms of depression. Negative events in your life can also precipitate depression.

As emphasized by cognitive behavioral therapists, your thoughts about such events lead you to become upset, but by altering such disabling thoughts you can alleviate depression.

> For psychotherapy to be effective for individuals with bipolar illness, it must foster increased self-awareness. It is most advantageous when it also helps a patient discover specific skills for problem solving and for coping with the complexity of life's everyday challenges.

Sadness and hurt are natural reactions to negative events in one's life. It is when negative feelings are out of proportion to the event that a depressed mood is triggered and maintained. It is a loss of self-esteem that leads to depression. Feeling that you are no good, that your worth has decreased, or that you are inadequate are just a few examples of decreased self-esteem. If you convince yourself that things will never get better and lose interest in even trying to improve your situation, then you are fostering and keeping that depression alive. While negative feelings are always an appropriate reaction to upsetting events, it is the conclusions you draw regarding such feelings and events that can foster depression.

Aaron Beck, a pioneer in the development of cognitive therapy, assumes that depressed people are subject to the "cognitive triad": feelings of negativism, pessimism, and helplessness about themselves, their world, and their future. These feelings derive from core patterns of distorted belief systems. To the degree that individuals lack awareness of their belief systems, these systems influence their daily thinking and are especially powerful during times of emotional stress.[2]

Core Beliefs

In cognitive behavior therapy, these core beliefs are called "schema." In a sense, they are the underlying philosophy one has about life. They serve as a lens, or a template, for information processing. We view, categorize, and make sense of all of our experiences according to these core beliefs. These beliefs influence all observations and interpretations of our experiences.

Examples of core beliefs include: I need to have everyone love me; I need to be perfect; I need to have, and should have, complete control over my life. These core beliefs, which are deeply rooted and often unconscious, predispose us to entertain thoughts that may actually foster negative moods, including depression. For example, when you operate from a deeply held core belief that any experience, short of perfection, is equal to a failure, it is easy to understand how you might automatically think: I am inadequate . . . I don't measure up . . . I am no good.

> Core beliefs are deeply rooted, often unconscious, and predispose us to entertain thoughts that may actually foster negative moods, including depression.

Cognitive therapy describes these kinds of thoughts as automatic. In a sense, they form our "automatic pilot," guiding us through the day. Cognitive behavior treatment for depression involves helping the patient become aware of these automatic thoughts as they occur. Automatic thoughts, while at times unconscious, are more accessible to one's actual awareness than more deeply unconscious core beliefs.

Self-Talk

Self-talk is conversation we have with ourselves, our internally voiced thoughts about others, the world around us, and ourselves. Everyone engages in self-talk whether at home, at work, in a car or in a store, interacting with loved ones, observing people on a bus, in the company of others, or alone. Some of us are more aware than others of these ongoing thoughts, and each of us varies in the amount of self-talk we engage in.

When we are busy and focused on an activity or very engaged with people, we are unaware of self-talk. In fact, we are living in an age in which we are increasingly bombarded by external stimulation that competes with our noticing self-talk. Our society so strongly encourages us to be active and productive that we often lack awareness of such dialogue. In many ways, our culture reinforces us to be overly concerned with the thoughts and attitudes of other people rather than to more fully identify and value our own way of thinking.

> Those living with bipolar illness are predisposed to operate on an automatic pilot that is constricted during depression and without limits during manic periods.

Throughout the day we all make decisions, some of which are based on thoughtful consideration while others are based on an internal automatic pilot. By this we mean that certain decisions and actions are made automatically without our seeming to pay them much attention. These decisions result from ideas that become our knee-jerk thoughts. Knee-jerk thoughts are rapid and immediate self-talk that usually is based on our core beliefs and influenced by distortions in thinking. We behave as if on automatic pilot. We have emotional reactions, make decisions, and take actions based on self-talk that may or may not be within our conscious awareness.

Those living with bipolar illness have emotional reactions, make decisions, and take action based on self-talk that is strongly influenced by the schema associated with depression or mania. These individuals are predisposed to operate on an automatic pilot that is constricted during depression and without limits during manic periods.

To better understand the idea of unconscious self-talk, it is helpful to understand how we focus our attention, shift attention, and attend to one area while ignoring another.

Selective Attention

Imagine that you are in a restaurant and actively engaged in talking with your best friend. At some point in your conversation, you hear two individuals at a nearby table mention the name of your company's CEO. Your interest is piqued. Although you had not been tuned in to that conversation before, now you're continuing to speak with your friend while paying attention to that intriguing discussion going on behind your back. You may even find yourself listening to the dialogue behind you rather than to your friend. This is an example of selective attention. We have the ability to choose to shift our focused attention to one of two separate conversations.

This same process occurs with our internal conversations. While we may be consciously aware of certain thoughts, other ideas may be taking place at a deeper, quieter level. It is only by attending to the unconscious self-talk that we can become more acutely self-aware and know the wider range of our thoughts and emotions.

Core beliefs, as previously illustrated, are based on distortions of thinking that may predispose us to entertain automatic thoughts grounded in faulty thinking. Core beliefs influence our thinking to the extent of guiding us to pay too much attention to some details while ignoring others. A core belief that you need to be perfect may frequently lead you to an automatic thought that you are a "failure" even if you make just one mistake at any given task. Core beliefs may similarly lead you to other distortions in information processing that reflect a negative focus.

The process of identifying automatic thoughts leads to identifying the core beliefs that underlie such thoughts. Cognitive behavioral

Examples of Distorted Thinking

Overgeneralization   A pattern of drawing a general rule or conclusion based on one or more isolated incidents and applying that rule or conclusion to related and unrelated situations.[3]

Example: "Since I wasn't accepted for that job, I'm convinced I shouldn't bother applying for those other positions."

Example: "If I'm depressed, it must be because I have bipolar illness."

Selective abstraction   Focusing on a detail of a situation and then conceptualizing the whole experience on the basis of that one detail.[4]

Example: "I'm sure I won't get that position. I made a mistake in that one answer."

Example: "If I get dry mouth with this medication, I need to discontinue taking it."

Dichotomous thinking   Thinking in extremes and labeling experiences in one of two extreme categories; for example, flawless or defective, saint or sinner.[5]

therapists utilize a wide variety of techniques to foster this process. Some therapists focus on shared discussion exploring the details of a person's experiences that may have preceded feelings of depression. The patient may be helped to identify specific situations and his reactions to them. He may be encouraged to explore his thoughts, his emotional reactions, observations, or other experiences related to the event in an effort to gain insight regarding automatic thoughts and core beliefs. For example, a patient may recall being ignored by her husband during dinner. Through shared discussion and her self-reflection, she may recognize automatic thoughts as conclusive regarding her experience. Automatic conclusions may include "He doesn't

Example: "If I'm not accepted for that position, I'm a failure."

Example: "If I don't feel comfortable with that therapist, I should give up therapy."

Discounting the positives   Focusing only on the negative aspects and discounting the positive aspects.[6]

Example: "I performed weakly in every part of the interview (when in fact I exhibited many strengths)."

Example: "I had one brief manic period during this past year. That proves I'm not getting better."

Labeling   Instead of viewing an incident as a mistake, applying a global label to oneself.[7]

Example: "What I said at the party was really foolish. . . . I'm just a jerk."

Example: "How could I have taken that medication while taking lithium. . . . I'm so stupid."

really love me," "I'm so boring" or, "I'm responsible for making this enjoyable." They may also suggest assignments between sessions that encourage the patient to increase his attention to events and specific thoughts which can be presented during the next meeting.

Other therapists may be highly structured in their approach. For example, as part of the initial assessment, the therapist may ask patients to complete questionnaires in order to identify their attitudes. One such questionnaire is the Dysfunctional Attitude Scale, an inventory that assesses attitudes such as vulnerability (asking for help is a sign of weakness), attraction/rejection ("I am nothing if a person does not love me."), and perfectionism ("My life is wasted unless I am a success.").[8]

Therapists might also ask their patients to keep a daily journal in an effort to identify thoughts that might help "turn up the volume" on quieter thoughts. Another approach is to have patients use forms to monitor their experiences; on the forms, they record the emotions, thoughts, and behaviors that accompany the experiences. These methods enable patients to develop more objective attitudes in assessing themselves.

"I encourage my clients to monitor their thoughts in a variety of ways," says Bernie Golden. "First, you might keep a journal that involves any ongoing narrative regarding specific experiences. Or, you may be helped to identify your thoughts by keeping a structured log." For example, such a log may include

- The date of some particular incident
- A description of the situation
- Any emotions surrounding the event (with a rating of their intensity)
- Automatic thoughts (rating the intensity)
- A rational response (rating the intensity)
- An outcome that includes a rating of the intensity of your belief in the automatic thought process in addition to the rating of the intensity of your emotion following the challenge of rational thinking

Therapists work with clients to develop skills that increase their capacity for self-reflection and, thereby, foster an increased awareness of their thoughts. Role-playing and discussion are useful tools. Through repeatedly asking themselves questions and identifying the content of their thoughts, clients increase their awareness of the distorted thinking that influences their thoughts and moods. Some therapists use cognitive therapy in combination with psychodynamic therapy. When these approaches are practiced together, they help the client identify the dynamics and patterns of past experiences that may have influenced the development of the client's core beliefs.

Case Study:
Moderate Depression and Cognitive Therapy

In his first cognitive therapy session, Matt, a 28-year-old lawyer, described how he had become increasingly depressed. While he did well professionally for the first two years after joining a law firm, in the past four months he had suffered setbacks, losing two significant cases. He also shared that, against his desires, a five-year relationship ended six months prior to his seeking treatment. Matt described feeling inadequate, weak, anxious, and depressed. Similarly, he reported difficulties in sleeping, a reduced appetite, and lethargy in attending to work and to activities that previously provided him pleasure. In addition, he reported increased social isolation over the past few weeks. Although Matt experienced no active suicidal ideation, he did have some fleeting ideas about welcoming "the end" if it were to occur.

> Through repeatedly asking themselves questions and identifying the content of their thoughts, clients increase their awareness of the distorted thinking that influences their thoughts and moods.

Matt evidenced a moderate level of depression. If it had been more severe, medication therapy might have been in order. Depressive thoughts can be paralyzing, and the tunnel vision of depression can hamper a severely depressed patient from receiving any measurable benefit from cognitive therapy. In a severely depressed state, a patient is sometimes unavailable to engage in the collaborative effort and process of standing back and observing his or her own thoughts. During this phase, medication therapy is usually an essential component of treatment.

In Matt's case, cognitive therapy helped alleviate his depression. In addition to therapy sessions, Matt kept a personal journal and adhered to a variety of structured exercises to identify those moments when he felt most depressed and what his thoughts were during those moments.

Through discussion of his journal entries and guided interventions in the sessions, Matt was helped to identify and clarify those automatic thoughts that coincided with and followed those depressed moments. In addition, by increasing his skills in recognizing his thought processes, he was able to identify the thoughts he had during meetings at his law firm. These automatic thoughts included: I need to be a senior partner in the firm by age 30 or I'm a failure; I'm feeling that my successes were just luck; I'm feeling completely inadequate.

Therapy helped Matt identify thoughts he had outside of work as well. He reported moments when he wanted to relax, but then quickly reconsidered because of the guilt he would feel over not working more productively on his cases. When he would so much as entertain the thought of seeking companionship, he automatically thought, "I will never love someone again as much as I loved Jane."

It took several sessions before Matt experienced being able to recognize, and appreciate, his "quiet" thoughts. He began to turn up the volume on his self-talk, something he had not attended to previously. In addition, Matt recognized the frequency of these thoughts. He became increasingly aware of how his thoughts influenced his experience of fear, tension, irritability, and depression. Later, he was in a better place to recognize some distortions in his thought processing that had led to his automatic thoughts. These included labeling, discounting the positives, selective abstraction, and overgeneralization.

> A challenging thought is one that offers an alternative by which we can more objectively gauge our expectations and conclusions. Through repetition, the challenging self-talk replaces the unrealistic thought and becomes a part of our automatic pilot.

The next step in Matt's treatment involved helping him to challenge these distortions with more objective thoughts. A challenging thought is one that offers an alternative by which we can more objectively gauge our expectations and conclusions. Through repetition, the challenging self-talk replaces the unrealistic thought and becomes a part of our automatic pilot.

A challenging thought is one that draws attention to the real world and illustrates how people actually behave. In focusing on more mature logic, we call attention to the realistic probability of things happening a certain way. Whereas unrealistic expectations may really be "wishes," the challenging thought is bound by reality.

In a way, this approach pits the objective reasoning part of us (the rational, mature, reasonable, parental, and nurturing part) against the unrealistic reasoning part of us (the part that creates distorted appraisals, has unrealistic expectations, and is impulsive and sabotaging). The objective reasoning part must be activated in treatment of any kind.

A challenging statement is often simple, both in wording and in its message. The more concise and basic the language, the more easily it becomes a part of our automatic internal dialogue and influences our expectations and conclusions. Cognitive therapy helped Matt develop challenges for each of his automatic thoughts, as outlined in table 2.

In the process of learning to challenge distorted thinking, we learn skills in self-soothing. This is a major part of effective change in the management of depression as well as other uncomfortable emotions. Therapy helped Matt develop challenging thoughts (that is, realistic thoughts to replace unrealistic thoughts) related to his sadness concerning the ending of his relationship. With further work, he became aware of core beliefs that served as the foundation for some of his automatic thoughts. The core beliefs he uncovered included "I need to be perfect at everything I do" and "I am not worthy of love."

These core beliefs predisposed Matt to the intensity and pervasiveness of his depression, which was precipitated by losing the legal cases and his relationship. After helping Matt identify the core beliefs, his therapist then worked with him to develop numerous challenges to these core beliefs. As stated previously, through repetition, these challenges are integrated as part of our automatic thoughts, thereby permitting change to occur at a deeper level.

To the degree that depressed individuals do not recognize thoughts based on distorted thinking, they are, in fact, prisoners of their thoughts. If distorted thoughts are not recognized as such, they go unchallenged and options for changing our mood or behavior seem unavailable. In severe depression, any hope for change is absent.

Table 2. Automatic Thoughts and Challenges

Automatic Thoughts	Challenges
"I need to be a senior partner in the firm by age 30 or I am a failure."	"What if I don't make it, what then?" "I am not my feeling." "I will still survive." "While I *wish* to be a partner, I do not *need* to be a partner."
"I'm feeling that my successes were just luck."	"Just because I feel that way does not make it so." "I would have had to have an extreme percentage of luck to win all those cases." "I studied for years to gain that knowledge and put in many hours of work to win those cases."
"I'm feeling completely inadequate. I'm a failure."	"I am not my feeling." "I've won ten of twelve cases!" "Disappointment makes me think that way."

An experience of futility at having an impact on oneself or on others and a sense that the condition is permanent are characteristic of depression. The consistent and enduring attitudes are hopelessness, helplessness, and despair.

Tunnel Vision and Depression

Kay Jamison describes the overwhelming influence of such thinking that formed the tunnel vision of her depressive periods. "My thinking, far from being clearer than a crystal, was torturous. I was used to my mind having analytic thought. Now, all of a sudden, my mind had turned on me: it mocked me for my vapid enthusiasms; it laughed at all of my foolish plans; it no longer found anything interesting or enjoyable or worthwhile. It was incapable of concentrated thought and turned time and again to the subject of death: I was going to die, what difference did it make?"[9]

Clearly, Jamison's thoughts became compelling and left little, if any, room to consider alternative attitudes. During those moments, she was a prisoner held captive by the compelling intensity of those despairing attitudes.

> To the degree that depressed individuals do not recognize thoughts based on distorted thinking, they are, in fact, prisoners of their thoughts.

Most individuals with severe depression need medication therapy to help reduce symptoms, including negative thinking that becomes a major aspect of depression. Judge Sol Wachtler, whose story appears in chapter 1, states that Prozac is what most helped him deal with his depression. While some research suggests gains without medication, most mental health professionals emphasize the use of medications as a major component of treatment of severe depression.

As medication can decrease the intense hold of depressive thinking, cognitive therapies can have their greatest impact in responding to mild and moderate levels of depression. It is during this phase of mood disorder that clients are more genuinely available to step back and observe their thoughts. In doing so, they gain increased freedom from their automatic pilots and, subsequently, gain more control of their moods and attitudes.

While not immediately apparent, those with mania can also be constrained by their thinking. Typically, we associate mania as boundless in energy and thought. In contrast to those with depression, people experiencing mania are often held hostage by their energy and impulses. In severe mania, the hostage element is especially notable for the lack of capacity to accurately assess the reality, safety, and/or appropriateness of their behavior. These individuals are compelled by thoughts that race and propel them into action, thoughts that reflect little or no restraint, and, in the extreme, thoughts dominated by a "logic" that lacks reality-based cause-and-effect thinking.

It is faulty thinking and the inability to control one's thoughts and activities that are most debilitating in severe mania. Core beliefs are often at the foundation of obsessiveness in mania. While on one level mania is associated with optimism, manic energy can fuel the obsessive actions that the individual in the manic cycle takes in response to underlying and predisposing core beliefs, such as "I *must* be perfect."

> In contrast to those with depression, people experiencing mania are often held hostage by their energy and impulses. In severe mania, the hostage element is especially notable by the lack of capacity to accurately assess the reality, safety, and/or appropriateness of their behavior.

While individuals who exhibit mania may be helped to identify automatic thoughts and distortions in thinking, those who experience low-level mania clearly have little motivation for such treatment. Automatic thoughts associated with mania may be overly optimistic and grandiose. Subsequently, these thoughts do not promote discomfort, which so often is the motivating force to seek treatment. Patients encountering more severe mania are even less available to stop and reflect on their thoughts. Individuals with mild depression and mania, however, as well as those in a more stable mood, can greatly benefit from coping skills therapy, another form of cognitive behavior therapy.

COPING SKILLS THERAPY

While cognitive restructuring involves attention to internal thoughts, coping skills therapy focuses on helping individuals alter the way they respond to external negative events. In this context, individuals learn to identify and alter thoughts, images, and actions that may help reduce the negative impact of such events.

Take the example of a person with bipolar illness who loses her job. Coping skills therapy can help her alter her thoughts, images, and actions by being responsive to her feelings regarding that loss—anxiety, frustration, hurt, and anger. In therapy, she can learn relaxation exercises to decrease her anxiety. Therapy can help her identify actions she can take to move on. It can also assist her in developing assertiveness skills or communication skills that will enable her to respond better to external stressors. Certainly, through coping skills therapy, she can identify how her illness may have contributed to her reactions to losing her job. The focus in this approach is on action, however.

In the case of someone with a predisposition for depression, coping skills provide alternative ways of responding to bad events. This helps prevent a spiraling sense of negativism from dominating how we feel, think, and act in response to loss. The goal of such therapy is not to eliminate the emotional reactions to loss, but rather to reduce their intensity by reducing the pervasiveness, longevity, and global quality of thoughts prompted by the loss. In this instance, some aspects of cognitive restructuring may be useful in conjunction with coping skills therapy.

> In the case of someone with a predisposition for depression, coping skills provide alternative ways of responding to bad events. This helps prevent a spiraling sense of negativism from dominating how we feel, think, and act in response to loss.

Clearly, coping skills are useful for those of us with bipolar illness. As with other forms of therapy, we can benefit most when we are in a stable mood. While such skills can be learned following upsetting events, it may be more effective to include coping skills therapy as part of a proactive approach toward mood stabilization.

PROBLEM-SOLVING THERAPY

Problem-solving therapy focuses on helping individuals learn processes that help them identify, discover, or invent a variety of effective or adaptive means of coping with specific problems encountered in everyday life.[10] In addition, problem solving processes help one select the most effective response from these choices. "A problem is defined as a life situation that demands a response for effective functioning, but for which no effective response is immediately available to the individual (or group) confronted with the situation."[11]

The solutions to any of these problems involve developing strategies to help individuals alter their environment and/or how they respond to their environment. Problem-solving therapy is most beneficial for individuals with bipolar illness when it is approached as a proactive rather than reactive program. Again, the best window of opportunity to learn such skills is during low-level depression or mania or a period of mood stability.

Each of us encounters a variety of problems in our daily lives. You may be confronted with a friend who is habitually late for scheduled meetings. When you brainstorm to arrive at alternative ways to respond to this situation, you are using problem-solving skills. Deciding on the advantages and disadvantages of the various ways of responding is another aspect of problem solving. As a result of engaging in problem solving, you might decide to learn and practice a coping strategy, such as assertiveness skills, so you can feel comfortable communicating to your friend how you are affected by his lateness. Or, you may choose not to spend time with this friend. Other possible solutions include scheduling your meeting ten minutes earlier than you would ideally want to meet, or bringing a book to read to give you something to do while you're waiting for your late friend.

In contrast, you could focus the problem solving on how you interpret his lateness. As a result of this work, you might decide to develop skills to monitor your predisposition to be self-critical (as reflected by self-doubt concerning the correct time of the meeting) or to interpret the lateness as a sign of rejection or lack of caring.

Problem-solving therapy helps the individual come up with a range of alternative responses to a situation. The client then judges each potential solution by considering four areas:

1. Problem resolution

2. Emotional well-being

3. Amount of time and effort required

4. Overall personal/social well-being[12]

The process of problem solving is dependent on a variety of skills that can be learned. Some cognitive behavioral therapists identify five key phases of problem solving:

1. General orientation

2. Problem definition

3. Generate alternatives

4. Decision making

5. Verification

General orientation refers to how we view problems in general. We can identify our general orientation by answering such questions as: "Do I take for granted that problems are a natural part of life?" or "Am I optimistic or pessimistic about problems and my ability to solve them?"[13]

Defining a problem involves stating it as a conflict between a goal and an obstacle preventing the achievement of that goal. Generating alternatives involves giving oneself permission to brainstorm, with an emphasis on not being self-critical and on listing as many alternatives as possible. Decision making entails weighing the advantages and disadvantages of the alternatives and deciding which ones to use. Finally, verification involves taking action and assessing the outcome.

Learning these skills offers those with bipolar illness (and others) an organized approach to dealing with problems that are invariably a part of daily life. The process of problem solving emphasizes resolution.

Cognitive therapy makes an important distinction between treatment that is problem focused and treatment that is emotion focused.[14] Problem-focused treatment emphasizes goals for changing the problem situation. In contrast, emotion-focused treatment emphasizes changing one's reactions to the situation in order to reduce the stress it arouses. In this case, treatment assists the individual in changing the "meaning" or appraisal of the situation, challenging automatic thoughts, reducing autonomic (physiological) arousal, and enhancing personal growth.

Self-management is another component of treatment that falls in the category of problem-solving skills. Self-management involves helping an individual identify strategies to maintain his practice of certain behaviors. A major premise of this approach is that the individual is available to observe, monitor, reflect on, or even initiate behavior. As part of a comprehensive program for manic-depression, self-management is an especially important component for regulating sleep, eating habits, exercise, nutrition, and other habits that promote stability and overall well-being.

> It is during the low level of depression or mania that an individual is most open to the development of habits of behavior and thinking that foster stability. To a great extent, the goal of practicing self-management skills during these periods is to make them a natural part of one's repertoire.

Once again, it is during the low level of depression or mania that an individual is most open to the development of habits of behavior and thinking that foster stability. To a great extent, the goal of practicing these skills during these periods is to make them a natural part of one's repertoire. Through continued rehearsal, one can gain the capacity to observe signs of escalating mania or depression. Through repeated monitoring, one can become more able to regulate relevant behaviors and/or seek support regarding them. Self-management involves self-monitoring, self-evaluation, and self-reinforcement.

TREATMENT COMPLIANCE

A major challenge in the treatment of bipolar illness is the lack of compliance with medication treatment and with psychotherapy. While some clients readily adhere to a medication regime that helps reduce the debilitating effects of bipolar illness, others refuse to take medication, take too little, determine their own dosage, or develop their own schedule for taking it. In a similar manner, some individuals with bipolar illness refuse psychotherapy or make minimal use of it.

Numerous factors contribute to a lack of compliance with both medication and psychotherapeutic treatment. Patients with severe depression may not be available to utilize such treatment. The intensity and pervasiveness of depressive thoughts and emotion compete with optimism and an openness to considering other thoughts. A patient's negative attitude about the treatment can also interfere with compliance. This is especially true when these attitudes are based on the same patterns of distorted thinking that fostered the depression in the first place. Examples of negative attitudes that obstruct compliance include:

"I feel controlled by the therapist if I do a journal, engage in self-reflection, monitor my thinking, or take medication."

This attitude may be related to core beliefs such as "I need to solve my problems by myself," and automatic thoughts such as "I am too emotionally weak to need help . . . I'm just too dependent!"

"I need a guarantee that it (the medication or therapeutic suggestion) will work."

This attitude may derive from a core belief that "I should never be disappointed" and over-generalization expressed by "If this medication does not work, I'm sure others will not work."

"I enjoy the emotional high when I am manic and don't want to give it up, even though I might have many negative consequences later."

This attitude may be based on selective attention.

"I am afraid of doing the exercises. Something bad will happen."

This may be an expression of core beliefs that "Change is not good."

"Nothing will change, and there are too many side effects."

This reaction may be derived from discounting the positives.

"I will lose my creativity, spontaneity, and my very personality if I take medication or engage in psychotherapy."

The core belief, "I should not have to experience uncertainty in order to get better," may underlie this attitude.

"I need to make these changes immediately."

This attitude may derive from a core belief that "When I want something to happen, it should and it should come quickly and easily."

Another obstacle to compliance is when individuals with bipolar illness focus only on the positive aspects of their manic episodes and minimize, deny, or ignore the overall impact of the illness. Such clients struggle with any real loss they may experience as a part of treatment and with any perceived loss which they may anticipate. They need help both in dealing with that loss and in recognizing that certain of their fears are not realistic.

SUMMARY

Psychotherapy is an invaluable component in the treatment of bipolar illness. Such treatment offers knowledge, understanding, and skills. Most significantly, psychotherapy fosters empowerment and addresses the difficult experience of facing life's challenges while living with bipolar illness.

Successful treatment depends on the ability to recognize and openly discuss all pertinent concerns as we have outlined above. This requires a trusting therapeutic relationship that allows a candid exploration of the underlying emotions, attitudes, and behaviors that compete with the attitudes and behaviors favorable to compliance.

Cognitive behavior therapy can help individuals with bipolar illness challenge distorted thoughts, learn self-monitoring techniques, develop coping strategies, and recognize and be able to manage the motivations that may compete or interfere with their overall improvement. The success of therapy depends on patient commitment to assuming an active role in the therapeutic process and the sharing of these concerns. Simultaneously, successful therapy requires a therapist who is aware of the issues surrounding medication and psychotherapeutic treatment for bipolar illness.

CHAPTER 6

The Prevention of Suicide in Bipolar Disorder

SUICIDE IS THE eighth leading cause of death in the United States and third in youth ages 15 to 19, resulting in more than 30,000 deaths each year. There is concern that the rate of suicide may be sharply increasing as a result of decreasing availability of treatment and bureaucratically managed care plans.[1]

Suicide is a major risk in people with bipolar disorder, and we are losing too many. As we have pointed out in previous chapters, early diagnosis and treatment, which results in a stabilization of the illness, is a basic approach to reducing suicidal risk. But in some instances, even treated patients may break through with symptoms of depression or mixed states of bipolar disorder. The accurate assessment and rapid treatment of these patients can be lifesaving. In this chapter, we will discuss the assessment of acute and chronic suicide risk in patients with bipolar disorder.

WHO IS AT GREATEST RISK AND WHEN?

Completed suicide is four times more frequent in men (5:1 in adolescents) than women, but two times more women than men attempt suicide. Of people who complete a suicide, 60 to 70 percent had talked to friends about it in the preceding six months. Statistics indicate that 8 to 25 suicide attempts are made for every suicide that is completed.

> *S*uicide is four times more frequent in men than women (5:1 in adolescents), but two times more women than men attempt suicide. Of people who complete a suicide, an estimated 60 to 70 percent had talked to friends about it in the preceding six months.

A recent study by Druss and Pincus in the *Archives of Internal Medicine* presented data on suicidal ideation and behavior. The study involved a standardized psychiatric interview from a sample of 7,589 adults (ages 17 to 39). The survey found 16.3 percent of the sample reported suicidal ideation, and 5.5 percent reported suicide attempts, in an otherwise healthy group. The incidences of suicidal ideation reported by those with one or more than one medical diagnosis respectively were 25 to 35 percent for suicidal ideation and 8.9 to 16.2 percent for reported suicide attempts. The risk for suicidal ideation increased 1.3-fold for patients with a diagnosis of major depression or alcoholism. Suicide attempts showed a 4-fold increased risk if the patient suffered from asthma or cancer. Suicides occur most commonly in the month of May, with April and June being the next most common times. Although most patients suffer more severely from depression between Thanksgiving and New Year's Day, it is in the burst of spring that suicide exerts its greatest threat.

Other factors that contribute to a high risk for attempting suicide are if the person is single, a white or Native American male, over the age of 50, or suffering from a chronic medical illness and viewing the future as a bleak one of continued poor health. Completed suicides occur more frequently among men over 65 years old.[2] However, the recent tripling of suicide rates in males ages 15 to 24 and doubling of the rate in young females has now established suicide as the third most common cause of death in 15- to 24-year-olds in

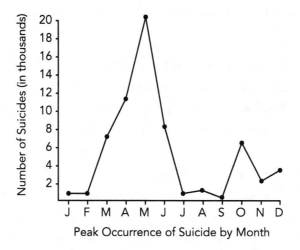

Figure 6.1—*Peak Occurence of Suicide by Month*
(Source: *Manic-Depressive Illness* by Frederick K. Goodwin and Kay R. Jamison, copyright 1990 by Oxford University Press, Inc. Used by permission of Oxford University Press, Inc.)

this country. Among college students, it is the second leading cause of death.

The mental health profession has been and still is reluctant to label children and adolescents with diagnoses traditionally applied to adults. Similarly, child psychiatrists are more reluctant to prescribe medications for children and adolescents. It is also difficult to distinguish bipolar illness from a variety of other conditions that may occur during what is viewed as normal adolescent turmoil. The behavior and emotions of children and adolescents can reflect a broad range of influences from disabilities, attention deficit disorder (ADD), delayed emotional development, and antisocial behavior.

In the bipolar population, statistics are high for suicide. Many studies show that approximately 15 percent of all people who suffer from manic-depression commit suicide. A recent English study, however, found the rate to be lower, about 6 percent.

> In the bipolar population, statistics are high for suicide. Approximately 6 to 15 percent of all people who suffer from manic-depression commit suicide, often early in illness.

Nick's Story

Nick Traina, son of author Danielle Steel, was one of the unfortunate statistics whose manic-depressive illness cost him his life. After her son's death, Steel wrote that if she had three wishes, they would be: "that he had never suffered from mental illness; that he were alive today; that someone had warned me, at some point, that his illness—manic-depression—could kill him."

Nick was different from other children. Severely troubled, he was a child of extremes. At age five, he drew pictures that depicted gore and violence and, by the age of eight, he had already begun to unravel. By 11, he was abusing over-the-counter medications to "still the demons."

This latter study found the risk was greatest early in the course of the illness. The difficulty in preventing suicide is compounded in this group by the difficulty in identifying the combination of specific factors that lead one individual with this diagnosis to cope and another to take his or her own life.

Psychosocial stressors are often responsible for triggering irrational and antisocial behavior in children or adolescents with bipolar disorder. In the case of the young, a child may not acquire a sufficient mastery of the challenges of adolescence and will thus be ill-prepared to move on. Even low-level stress (let alone mental illness) can be painful and overwhelming for teenagers as they face the increasingly complex tasks of maturation. While such stresses are common to many, the presence of clinical depression, substance abuse, significant anxiety, and/or a history of conduct disorder or impulsiveness can create a vulnerability to suicidal behavior.

Early diagnosis and treatment can help prevent a disaster. Effective treatments are currently available to help stabilize mood disor-

"Confusion has me strung out and desperate," said Nick. "My whole world is made of disillusion and pity, nothing more than a mirage, transparent, nonexistent. I reached out to try and touch my soul, but it was gone. I lost it somewhere. I am a scared little boy, and I don't know where to run. My little boy legs won't carry me much farther. I am weak when I always thought I had strength. My feet are in the air, my head is on the ground. Reality has set me spinning. I thought I could get up but there was more to it than that and I asked myself . . . where is my mind?"[3]

After three suicide attempts, Nick Traina took his life on the fourth.

ders so that the millions who suffer from bipolar disorder can regain, and maintain, a fulfilling and productive life.

SUICIDE RISK FACTORS

Table 3 shows common risk factors for suicide in patients with bipolar disorder, depressive disorders, alcoholism, schizophrenia, and borderline personality disorder.

If any suicidal thoughts or behaviors become apparent, or if relatives even suspect that the patient is thinking about suicide, the treating psychiatrist should be called immediately. It is possible that hospitalization may be required. As with the development of chest pains in a heart patient, the development of suicidal feelings or several other risk factors in a person with bipolar illness indicates the need for immediate expert evaluation.

Although studies have identified the risk factors listed in the table in patients with the psychiatric disorders, it should be recognized that

Table 3. Acute and Chronic Risk Assessment Factors for Suicide and Suicide Attempt

Risk Factors	Acute Risk (hours to weeks)	Chronic Risk (months to years)	Treatment Response	
			(hours to days)	(weeks to months)
High Risk Diagnoses				
Bipolar		+		+
Major Depression		+		+
Schizophrenia		+		+
Alcoholism-depression		+		+
Borderline disorder with depression		+		+
Other Risk Factors				
Suicide ideation (past)		+		
Suicide impulse and plan	+			
Past attempt		+		
Recent attempt	+/-	+		
Severe psychic anxiety	++		+	
Panic attacks	++		+	
Severe agitation	++		+	

Risk Factors	Acute Risk (hours to weeks)	Chronic Risk (months to years)	Treatment Response	
			(hours to days)	(weeks to months)
Impulsivity	++	++	+	+
Recent alcohol abuse	++	+	+	
Past drug or alcohol abuse		+		
Global insomnia	++	+/-	+	
Severe anhedonia	+			+
Psychosis		+		+
Recent loss (relationship support, job)		+		
Discharge from psychiatric hospital within 6 to 12 months	+	+/-		
Male > 65		++		
Male		+		
Living alone		++		
No child <18 at home		++		

+ some risk   ++ high risk   +/- possible risk

even seasoned experts cannot accurately predict a suicide in any given individual. The presence of risk factors suggests the individual may be in a high-risk group of patients at the time observed. An evaluation followed by appropriate treatment should be obtained for any person displaying these high-risk features.

> The risk of suicide in bipolar disorder is highest during the de-pressive phase or during episodes of dysphoric mania.

The most common methods of suicide appear to be the most violent: death by shooting (58 percent) or hanging. Moreover, violent suicides are typically carried out in settings where there is little chance of being rescued.[4]

The lifetime risk of suicide in bipolar disorder is about 15 percent, approximately 1 percent of such patients per year. As noted above, a recent English study reported a lower long-term rate of 6 percent, but stressed the fact that suicide tended to occur early in the course of illness. Although some clinicians believe that the risk is higher with bipolar disorder than with unipolar depression, most studies show that the risk is the same. There is some evidence that the state of dysphoric mania (occurring in either bipolar type) and bipolar II disorder may carry a higher suicide risk than other forms of bipolar disorder. The risk of suicide in bipolar disorder is highest during the depressive phase or during episodes of dysphoric mania (see chapter 2).

CAN SUICIDE RISK BE DETECTED IN TIME TO HELP PREVENT A SUICIDE?

Unfortunately, it is not generally possible even for mental health professionals to accurately predict an individual suicide. That said, it is important to learn to recognize the features that place a person in a high-risk category and to get an evaluation by a trained expert. People who take their own lives may have had depression or bipolar disorder with suicidal ideas for some time. Suicidal thoughts result from hopelessness and recurrent severe anxiety that can eventually produce intolerable "psychic pain" that cries for relief. In ruminating about suicide, some patients even develop a specific suicide plan. Criteria for high-risk must be further examined and, where indicated, an individual must receive treatment which may include hospitalization. The following questions are most useful in determining a patient's suicide risk:

Do you feel hopeless about life, or sometimes feel like life is too painful to continue living?

Are you suffering from constant worry, anxiety attacks, and/or the inability to sit still?

Are you fearful of the future, and do you have episodes of pacing?

What are your reasons for living at this point?

Do you have any thoughts of dying or of ending your life?

Have you attempted suicide in the past, or have you acted self-destructively on impulse?

Do you have a suicidal plan?

Do you have the means to carry it out (e.g., a gun, a high balcony)?

Communicated suicidal ideation—vocalized thoughts, such as, "I wish I was dead," or, "I won't take this any longer"—and prior suicide attempts are standard high-risk indicators. Suicidal communications prior to an attempt are much more commonly imparted to family and friends than to doctors or mental health professionals. Anyone who receives such a communication should report it immediately to someone who can help.

The classic studies of Eli Robins concluded that approximately 70 percent of patients who committed suicide had mentioned the thought during the year prior to their actual death. Robins found 60 percent of patients communicated suicidal ideation to spouses, 50 percent to friends, and only 18 percent communicated to helping individuals such as doctors and counselors.[5]

That means that if a loved one, relative, or friend talks to you about suicidal thoughts, that person may not be leveling with their doctor or therapist about such thoughts. If there is evidence of preoccupation, a suicide plan, or talk of lethal means (such as a gun, hanging, jumping, or carbon monoxide from a car), take it seriously and consider it an emergency situation.

> Of those who expressed suicidal thoughts in the year prior to their actual death, 60 percent communicated suicidal ideation to spouses, 50 percent to friends, and only 18 percent communicated to helping individuals such as doctors and counselors.

Recent studies have shown that, before taking their lives, people frequently deny any suicidal ideation or intent to commit suicide when asked by their doctor or other professional. Therefore, it can be naive to dismiss suicide as a potential risk simply because a patient denies suicidal ideation, especially if other risk factors are present. Some patients who have made a decision to end their lives will deny any suicidal intent, but show other risk factors. A careful clinical evaluation can result in lifesaving treatment; many patients have been lost because this was not available to them.

A history of suicide attempts, especially over time, increases the risk of suicide. This is supported by follow-up studies of patients who attempted suicide; these studies found that 7 to 12 percent completed suicide over a 10-year period.[6,7] Any history of attempted suicide is important to know when evaluating a depressed individual. A positive family history of suicide also increases suicide risk.[8]

The presence of impulsiveness, a trait that is frequently apparent in individuals with a history of alcohol or substance abuse and certain personality disorders (antisocial personality, borderline personality, and rapid cycling or mixed states of bipolar disorder), adds another high-risk factor for suicidal behavior when depression is also present.

The Role of Anxiety in Suicide Risk

In recent studies we have found that severe psychic anxiety, often of a ruminative type (see below), and the occurrence of panic attacks and agitation are also associated with acute high risk in the presence of depression.[9]

When panic attacks occur together with the hopelessness that can accompany depression, some patients feel that suicide is their only way out. In a study of 954 hospital inpatients, followed for over 10 years, 62 percent of those who killed themselves within 1 year of evaluation had panic attacks together with major depression. We know that panic attacks occur in approximately 25 to 30 percent of all patients with major depressive disorders. The presence of total or global insomnia, the inability to concentrate, severe anhedonia (the inability to experience usual interest and pleasure), and recent moderate alcohol abuse are also high-risk indicators.

Anxiety may present in several different forms, such as the ruminative anxiety mentioned above. Ruminative anxiety is severe, pervasive, and recurrent anxiety that dominates a person's thoughts over a problem

> When panic attacks occur together with the hopelessness that can accompany depression, some patients feel that suicide is their only way out.

that anyone might worry about to some degree, such as financial concerns, possible legal problems, or problems with relationships. The anxiety becomes pathological when the particular problem consumes almost all of an individual's attention and is out of proportion to the actual danger of harm. All other issues become secondary when the central theme in a patient's mind is otherwise focused. For instance, a person may become persistently worried over a minor legal

A Suicide Prevention Pact

In *Night Falls Fast,* Kay Jamison reveals an agreement she made with her friend Jack: "We were talking about suicide and making a blood oath. . . . We both had manic-depressive illness and, despite the better and often expressed judgment of others, had a tendency to stop taking our lithium."

Their pact: if one of them felt suicidal, that person would contact the other and a plan of action to prevent the suicide would be enforced immediately. Their well-meaning intentions were not carried

violation or become concerned that he is suffering from a life-threatening disease such as cancer even before there is clear evidence. There is no escaping this fear, and the patient is unable to focus on anything else.

Some unfortunate individuals seem plagued by common worry over a lifetime. However, when someone develops a new pervasive, severe anxiety, especially when there is evidence of depression—such as social withdrawal, poor sleep, or loss of appetite—it is then not the topic of concern that is most important. It is the inescapable, fearful preoccupation combined with the hopelessness that accompanies depression, that is the major threat. As President Roosevelt said at the onset of World War II, "the only thing we have to fear, is fear itself."

Another form of anxiety is the occurrence of panic attacks superimposed on depression. Panic attacks, especially those connected with depression, are associated with an increased risk of suicide attempts. Depression associated with panic attacks, in contrast to depression alone, increases the risk of suicide within weeks to a few months. A high level of anxiety was found to be the most important short-term predictor of suicide, and perhaps the most treatable one, in a recent study.[10]

Some people have repeated panic attacks without depression. This condition is often diagnosed as panic disorder. The attacks are of a out, however. Many years later, Jamison's friend put a gun to his head and ended his life.

"Although shaken by Jack's suicide, I was not surprised by it," wrote Jamison. "Nor was I surprised that he had not called me. I, after all, had been dangerously suicidal myself on several occasions since our [pact was made] and certainly had not called him. Nor had I even thought of calling. Suicide is not beholden to an evening's promises, nor does it always hearken to plans drawn up in lucid moments and banked in good intentions."[11]

sudden onset and may occur in a stressful situation, in a crowd, while flying, or "out of the blue," as when someone is woken from sleep by a panic attack. Panic attacks are characterized by heart palpitations, a rapid (>100 beats/minute) pulse, and, often, acute difficulty in breathing or a feeling of not being able to get enough air. Chest pain, leading to fear of a heart attack, and feelings of being on the verge of fainting, losing control, and going "crazy" frequently also occur. Panic attacks can be manifested by angry outbursts or even sudden diarrhea. Suicide attempts have been observed with increased frequency in individuals with panic attacks.

A third form of severe anxiety state is agitation. Although often associated with severe psychic anxiety, agitation is also demonstrated by physical restlessness (pacing, the inability to sit still) and sometimes by moaning, shouting, or angry outbursts. Patients might express the feeling of being about to "jump out of their skin." Someone suffering this kind of anxiety may seem inconsolable. Agitated states can come and go quite abruptly, but may be persistent, or recurrent, in a person with ongoing symptoms of depression.

Immediate treatment for anxiety attacks is crucial in the depressed patient. The reduction of severe anxiety symptoms and agitation can reduce suicide risk even though the depression may take longer to

> Frequently, people assume an anxious, agitated person is better only to have the same state recur with tragic results after the "improved" person is left to manage alone.

respond to treatment. Several medications can quickly reduce anxiety, but the patient must be observed and the treatment continued; anxiety symptoms may recur rapidly once medication has worn off or the reassuring presence of a supportive person is no longer there if the depression has not been successfully treated. Frequently, people assume an anxious, agitated person is better, only to have the same state recur with tragic results after the "improved" person is left to manage alone.

WHAT CAN BE DONE TO PREVENT SUICIDE?

Suicide invariably induces a mixture of guilt and anger in friends and loved ones. In some cases, the suicide occurs even after every possible effort was made to help; nothing could have prevented it. When people become depressed, they often become less communicative and more socially withdrawn. It is common for a person, just prior to attempting suicide, to act as if no special problems are present, misleading loved ones and even expert clinicians.

Some people with severe depression often appear markedly improved just before committing suicide. Some, though clearly distressed, refuse treatment after deciding that their situation is hopeless or because they want to avoid the stigma of admitting a need for treatment. Other high-risk individuals reject help even more overtly, pushing away everyone's efforts to help.

Case Study: From Suicidal to Successful

Daniel, in his early 40s, was undergoing treatment consisting of lithium and psychotherapy. He was recovering from episodes of mania that had resulted in the loss of his job and previous career.

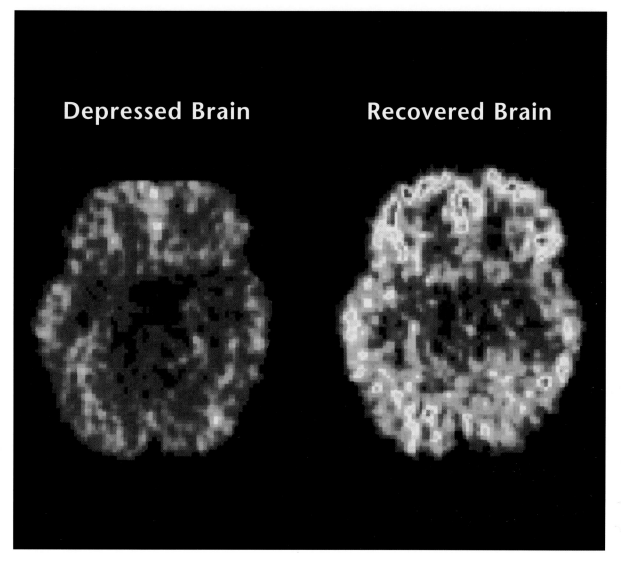

Depressed Brain **Recovered Brain**

(From Mark George, Terence Ketter, and Robert Post, Biological Psychiatry Branch, NIMH, Bethesda, Maryland, courtesy of Frederick K. Goodwin, M.D.)

PET scans (positron emission tomography) of the brain of a patient during depression and after recovery from depression. The colors in the scans correspond to glucose metabolic rates (which indicate activity of the neurons), with the lowest rates associated with the coolest end of the color spectrum (blue) and the highest rates with the warmest (red). If an area that normally reflects higher rates (red, yellow, or green) shows up blue on the scan, it implies that the neurons in that region are impaired in their function. The image made during a depressive episode (left) is dark, mostly blue, whereas the image created after treatment with medication (right) has more green, yellow, and red, showing that the activity of the neurons has normalized. See Imaging Studies, page 67.

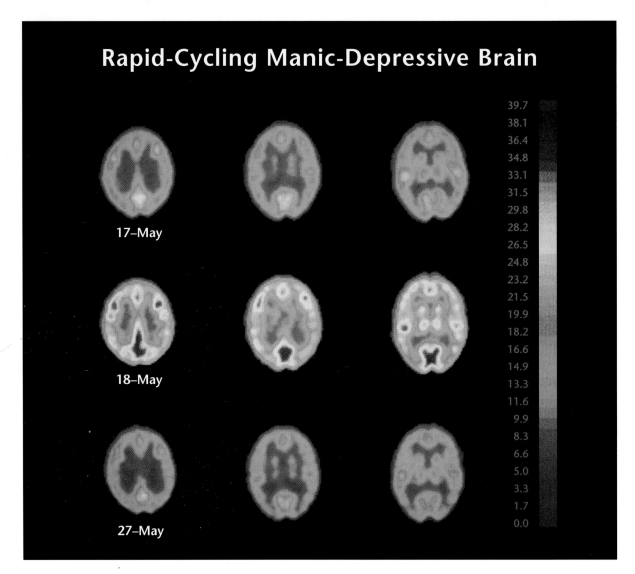

Rapid-Cycling Manic-Depressive Brain

17–May

18–May

27–May

| 39.7 |
| 38.1 |
| 36.4 |
| 34.8 |
| 33.1 |
| 31.5 |
| 29.8 |
| 28.2 |
| 26.5 |
| 24.8 |
| 23.2 |
| 21.5 |
| 19.9 |
| 18.2 |
| 16.6 |
| 14.9 |
| 13.3 |
| 11.6 |
| 9.9 |
| 8.3 |
| 6.6 |
| 5.0 |
| 3.3 |
| 1.7 |
| 0.0 |

(Image and text adapted from Baxter et al., 1985. Reprinted with permission from Oxford University Press.)

PET scans of the brain of a drug-free rapid-cycling manic-depressive patient. The images in the top row were made when the patient was depressed. The second row shows the identical planes scanned the next day, when the patient had become manic. The third row shows scans taken 10 days later when the same patient was again depressed. Impairment of metabolic function is expressed in the symptoms of clinical depression, such as slowed thought, lack of energy, loss of spontaneity, poor concentration, problems making decisions. In a manic state the metabolism of certain areas is increased at a supra-normal rate, correlating with increased energy, rapid thinking, rapid speech, decreased sleep, and hyperactivity. The scans show that this brain is in an abnormal metabolic state (either decreased or increased metabolic function) when the patient is in a depressed or manic state. See Imaging Studies, page 67.

While recovering and trying to begin a new career, he encountered major financial pressures and uncertainties. Despite his prior improvement, Daniel experienced a breakthrough depression related to this stress. Associated with the depression and financial worry, he also developed severe and intolerable anxiety attacks that increased in frequency and severity. All of this progressed to the point where he could no longer see the way out of his dilemma or tolerate the pain of his persistent anxiety. He purchased a gun and went off to a secluded place to take his life. After test-firing the gun, however, he decided to make one final attempt to get help before ending his life.

Daniel called his psychiatrist who saw that this was an emergency and hospitalized him at once. Daniel received antianxiety medication to control his overwhelming anxiousness, and started on antidepressant medication as well. Antidepressants commonly take from one to four weeks to lift a severe depression.

The antianxiety medication relieved his severe anxiety even though he still was plagued by financial problems.

Of the experience, Daniel said: "I felt overwhelmed. With the constant feeling of impending doom, I could see no way out. I couldn't stand the pain. Death seemed like the only relief from intolerable pain and failure. Then, when my anxiety decreased I began to see some long-term solutions to my very real problem. I realized it wasn't a life-and-death issue, and that I could work my way out of it."

Within two days, Daniel was discharged from the hospital, his condition markedly improved. With continued supportive treatment and medication, he gradually turned his life around and has since found a new and meaningful career helping others.

The Importance of a Strong Support System

Lincoln's story (see sidebar) is historical proof of the effectiveness and importance of surrounding a severely depressed and suicidal person with concerned, supportive, and giving friends. It appears that Lincoln's friends played a major role in his recovery, thereby permitting

Suicidal Tendencies: The Case of Abraham Lincoln

In *The Inner World of Abraham Lincoln,* biographer Michael Burlingame depicts the period in the young Lincoln's life when he was rejected by a woman he had hoped to marry and was consumed by serious financial problems. Moreover, he had a childhood history of maternal loss and physical abuse. These factors added to his vulnerability at a difficult period in his life and caused him to suffer severe depression and become preoccupied with suicide.

Lincoln's friends were so concerned that they literally moved in and stayed up with him day and night, after removing knives and guns from his presence. He remained agitated, spoke as if delirious, and was sleepless, with recurrent suicidal impulses. His friends maintained a constant vigil for a week or more until the crisis abated. Later, a friend invited Lincoln to live in his lodgings and paid his daily expenses as well as his law school tuition.

the man described by a friend as "the most ambitious man in the world" to express his talents on the nation's behalf. This is a prime example of what can be done to prevent suicide.

In Lincoln's case, however, he made known his distress to his friends and accepted their help. In some ways, the severity of his state, which rendered him helpless, may have made it easier for his friends to come to his rescue. They could be empathic, and he was in no position to resist the help offered. This is not always the case.

In many instances, people hide hopelessness, inner turmoil, and anxiety from friends and loved ones and even deny the existence of these emotions. The hopelessness that is intrinsic to suicidal depression often leads the person to reject help, especially treatment. It is as if the suicidal patient cannot tolerate one more disappointment or failure, such as the possible failure of efforts to improve what is experienced as a hopeless situation.

Gradually, Abraham Lincoln recovered and, despite other disappointments and depressive recurrences, was able to serve as the sixteenth president of the United States. Lincoln held the nation together during the grave crisis of the Civil War—not bad for someone "weak" enough to suffer suicidal depression!

Throughout his life, Abraham Lincoln exhibited many signs of continued high risk for suicide, including frequent recurrences of severe melancholic depression and suicidal ideation.

How did Lincoln survive well enough to be able to manifest such strength in the service of our nation? What enabled him to get through the periods of high suicide risk when medical and psychological treatment was unavailable? What seemed to be a major factor, as depicted in this biographical sketch of Lincoln, was his capacity to attract empathic and helpful friends and, most important, to accept their help in times of crisis.[12]

Depression narrows a person's vision of any positive alternatives. Any new direction, such as treatment, is viewed as just another source of uncertainty, pain, and failure. The obliteration of consciousness along with feelings of responsibility, torturous anxiety, failure, and guilt becomes a desired goal.

Often, the person experiences a fleeting vestige of hope regarding therapeutic treatment and its positive direction, but the sirens that sing of relief from all of life's psychic pain and self-hate are very seductive. Uncanny as it may seem, patients often appear suddenly and dramatically improved just before their suicide.

Talking with patients after a medically serious suicide attempt, one is struck by the

> The hopelessness that is intrinsic to suicidal depression often leads the person to reject help, especially treatment. It is as if the suicidal patient cannot tolerate one more disappointment or failure.

sense of peace and calm derived from the apparent freedom from all anxieties and criticism that the decision to commit suicide can create. What seems pitiful is that people die not realizing that it is possible to attain a similar state without having to exchange their conscious life to achieve it. Unfortunately, people often cannot see beyond the distortions imposed by their state of depression.

Demoralization Versus Clinical Depression

We frequently confuse a state of demoralization with clinical depression. People can try hard, do all the "right" things, be a "good" person, persevere, and still fail in their efforts or be struck down by some unexpected occurrence, such as an illness, tragic accident, or natural disaster. People often feel demoralized in such situations—beaten down, sad, and wanting to give up. They may even develop a clinical depression in response to these adverse events. But if they persist and fate finally rewards them, as God finally stopped testing Job, things begin to turn positive and life, once again, becomes happy.

> *The deeply depressed state of mind, all pervasive as it seems to the sufferer, can be completely lifted and held at bay by successful treatment. Doctors see this happen many times, and it is an amazing miracle to behold.*

In the case of a clinical depression, no possibility of redemption seems to exist. Clinically depressed people no longer experience success as positive. They view every occurrence, positive or negative, as having some fearful implication without any positive outcome even imaginable. The clinically depressed person on the verge of suicide can anticipate only further suffering and failure.

Even more problematic is that this mind state is not always continuous, but may alternate with some moments of distraction, during which the anxiety and suffering cease temporarily only to return again. Intermittent self-destructive impulses are the most frightening because of their unpredictability. A chronic negative state with its terrible predictability is sometimes easier to tolerate than attaining a glimmer of hope, only to be again plunged into fearful despair. Depression that views suicide as a solution is fueled by suffering—psychic pain colored by the fear and anticipation of increasing, uncontrollable, interminable pain. Is it any wonder that the surcease of death becomes attractive to a mind in this state?

We are all either prisoners or beneficiaries of our outlooks and attitudes, which determine how we experience life. We can all learn to endure pain with the anticipation of a better future. Depression can negatively distort a person's entire outlook; yet this state of mind, all pervasive as it seems to the sufferer, can be completely lifted and held at bay by successful treatment. Doctors see this happen many times, and it is an amazing miracle to behold.

SUICIDE: A PERMANENT SOLUTION TO A TEMPORARY PROBLEM

Depression distorts the problems of the afflicted into a never-ending state of suffering from which death seems the only relief. If patients survive suicidal impulses, however, they may regain their will to live.

One such case involved a man who hiked into the woods with full intent of ending his life. In an attempt to portray his suicide as an accident, he placed his rifle on a log, pointing the firearm at his chest. As he leaned over to pull the trigger, the rifle moved and accidentally discharged. Although the man was seriously wounded in the thigh, he crawled on his hands and knees for two miles, through deep snow, to get help.

This example clearly illustrates the will to survive if a person is able to get beyond the point of suicidal crisis. After that, the human instinct for self-preservation often reasserts itself.

Of course, in an untreated bipolar disorder or major depression, the hopelessness, pain, and suicidal wishes are likely to recur.

When depression is lifted by appropriate treatment, another problem has been solved. In the presence of depression, there is no way out, and it seems certain that more suffering and failure can only become more intolerable. It is difficult to imagine if you haven't been there, by experience or through empathy. Many people are reluctant to entertain the possibility that with free will (the ability to control one's own thoughts), the view of the world can become so negatively distorted. That is, to most of us who have never experienced a clinical depression and hopelessness, it is difficult to conceive of not being able to overcome this state with one's own efforts as we do in "normal" down states or life disappointments.

A doctor told a patient who did not respond to a series of treatment efforts that if he could just hang on and stay alive, the doctor was sure he would get better. A new treatment approach was finally successful and the patient returned to a normal state. The patient subsequently confided to the doctor, "I didn't believe you for one minute when you told me I could get better, but you were so persistent in trying to help me that I decided you either believed what you were saying or you were delusional. Your refusal to quit made me decide not to kill myself, and to stick around to see what would happen."

IMPLICATIONS FOR MANAGED CARE

Managed care criteria for predicting suicide, such as a requirement for expressed suicidal threats or a recent suicide attempt, are often inadequate for the assessment of suicide risk and the need for hospital care. Severe agitation and anxiety, panic attacks, and global insomnia may be considered insufficient indicators of the need for hospitalization if the patient denies suicidal ideation or has not attempted suicide previously.

The physician must be able to evaluate a patient without restriction by a managed care "protocol," which sometimes seems to override the clinical judgment of the doctor. When managed care plans disqualify patients from receiving coverage for psychiatric services on an inpatient basis, doctors frequently are at a loss to find alternative solutions for their patients. Not only does this exacerbate a patient's already high level of anxiety, but insufficient medical coverage also leads to lower levels of care. Suicidal patients may not get the care they require.[13]

An important caveat for supportive friends and relatives is that even a severely depressed patient may experience some transient hope after first seeing a skilled physician or counselor. When improvement is not immediate, the patient may feel disappointed that no miracle turnaround occurred. Profound hopelessness, cynicism, and recurrent anxiety can rapidly supplant transient hope following this disappointment. The risk of suicide can be very high at this time.

> *When managed care plans disqualify patients from receiving coverage for psychiatric services on an inpatient basis, doctors frequently are at a loss to find alternative solutions for their patients.*

It is important to stress that improvement may take time. Any first attempt at treatment, or the first medication tried, may need to be changed or modified before the best treatment is found. Hope is a fragile state in the mind of a clinically depressed person, and hope can turn into hopelessness in the absence of immediate success, especially if the patient is not given realistic expectations of treatment.

SUMMARY

Preventing suicide is not easy. First, you have to sense when a person with depression is in a state of immediate risk. Once that has been determined, the person should never be left alone until they have been examined by a professional and possibly hospitalized. If they can be induced to get help, it is wise to communicate with the professional about available options.

Offering a patient support until improvement has gradually occurred is very important. Be suspicious of dramatic recovery: When a

Preventive Measures for Suicide

The National DMDA lists the following recommendations for preventing the suicide of a family member, friend, or other person:

Take seriously the person's condition.

Stay calm, but don't under-react.

Involve other people. Don't try to handle the crisis alone or jeopardize your own health or safety. Call 911, if necessary.

Contact the person's psychiatrist, therapist, crisis intervention team, or others who are trained to help.

Express concern. Let the patient talk about suicidal thoughts without loved ones appearing to convey shock and condemnation. Give concrete examples of what leads you to believe the person is close to suicide. If this understanding is conveyed to the patient, then he or she may feel less guilty about possessing such suicidal thoughts.

Listen attentively. Maintain eye contact. Use body language, such as moving close to the person or holding his or her hand, if it is appropriate.

patient seems to rebound too quickly, it may indicate that they have given up, decided to commit suicide, and are pretending to be improved. Gradual recovery over days is much more reliable. Even then, sudden setbacks can occur. Remember the case of Abraham Lincoln, and how the sustained support of friends got him past his suicidal crisis.

You cannot prevent suicide in some instances. Even professionals can't always accurately predict, or prevent, a suicide. What you can do is try to recognize a high-risk period and stay with the patient or get someone else to stay until he or she is safe. Do not leave a person alone in a high-risk state. Also remove all firearms and other dangerous weapons and substances. Don't just think about it. Act! If you do

Ask direct questions. Inquire whether the person has a specific plan for suicide. Determine, if possible, what method of suicide the person is thinking about.

Acknowledge the person's feelings. Be empathetic, not judgmental. Do not relieve the person of responsibility for his or her actions, however.

Reassure. Stress that suicide is a permanent solution to temporary problems. Insist that the problem can be helped, even if past attempts have failed. Provide realistic hope. Remind the person that things can get better if the right help is made available. Stress that you will help them find effective treatment.

Don't worry about confidentiality! Confidentiality is secondary to a life-and-death situation. Don't hesitate to speak with the person's doctor in order to protect that person.

Do not leave the person alone, if possible, until you are sure that he or she is in the hands of competent professionals.

your best, and that is all anyone can be expected to do, you may save somebody's life.

Those who have previously attempted suicide and/or have a family history of suicide should take the following preventive measures:

- Be informed. Educate yourself through books, lectures, support groups, and consult with your local advocacy chapters (see the appendix, "Resources for Information").

- Contact your psychiatrist, therapist, crisis intervention team, or others who are trained to help.

- Ask for written information on all drugs you take, and be on the alert for any side effects.

CHAPTER 7

The Stigma of Mental Illness

STIGMA REFERS TO being characterized as deviant, flawed, limited, undesirable, or not measuring up in some way. When associated with mental illness, stigma is based on the view that such disorders reflect a weakened genetic strain, flawed heredity chain, weakness in character, purposeful malingering, lack of self-control, and/or immoral behavior.

HISTORY OF THE STIGMA OF MENTAL ILLNESS

Historically, stigma has been associated with mental illness as a chronology of collective understanding and attitudes toward individual will, responsibility, human behavior, and personality. Fear, ignorance, and shame have largely informed this history.

For centuries, mental illness was associated with mysticism and theology. Those who evidenced bizarre behavior were often thought to be influenced by the spirit world or by the forces of evil. In contrast, individual responsibility was emphasized when those with mental illness were viewed as having been sinful or as having lost faith in God. While sometimes sought out for having useful knowledge, those who evidenced bizarre behavior most often became victims of stigma and were both marginalized and ostracized.[1]

In ancient Greece, those with mental illness were often shunned or locked up. While explanations of mental illness were based mostly on beliefs regarding religion or magic, the Greeks were also the first to view mental illness as based on a physical disease. Hippocrates viewed epilepsy, melancholia, post-partum psychosis, and hysteria as medical illnesses rather than effects of divine influence.[2] In general, the illness was viewed as caused by the gods. While this explanation served to reduce some of the stigma, those with mental illness were still associated with shame and humiliation.[3]

Historically, frightening developments in the human condition were attributed to punishment by the gods. People found it comforting to blame the victim when facing tragedy. In biblical times, when friends of the long-suffering Job could find no other plausible explanation for the inexplicable tragedies that struck him, they blamed him, despite the fact that Job had lived a moral life.

During the Middle Ages people regarded symptoms of mental illness as evidence of communication between the afflicted individual and good or evil gods and spirits, often viewing sufferers as possessed by the devil. Witch-hunts and the burning of witches reflect the extreme consequence of such attitudes.

The extermination of those with mental illness during the Holocaust is another heinous response to stigma coupled with scapegoating. The wedding of mental illness and stigma has also been evidenced in countries that label dissidents as being emotionally disturbed, when, in fact, they may simply disagree with state politics.

Public reaction to mental illness is greatly influenced by a general lack of knowledge. The consequence of this ignorance is public fear, which has served historically to exacerbate the shame experienced by the afflicted and their loved ones. The stigma associated with mental disorders has, unfortunately, not abated.

Despite the ongoing stigma, efforts to teach public awareness while finding new ways of treating mood disorders continue to advance. These efforts have helped reduce fear and ignorance while paving the way for a more compassionate, humane, and realistic response to one of life's most complex challenges.

It is no surprise that the stigma of mental illness has been very strong in Western culture because our society places a high value on self-control, free will, and individual responsibility. Our society also expects us to exert self-control over our feelings and behavior. It is not difficult to see how these values, coupled with ignorance, have led to the public view of mental illness as a sign of character weakness.

This attitude may be especially prevalent toward individuals with bipolar illness. Those living with this disorder demonstrate wide variability in functioning, from healthy and "normal" to psychotic. A person's capacity to function in a normal manner may lead observers to conclude that weakness in willpower and self-control is responsible when that person "loses control." The fact that many symptoms of low-level mania are positive and fall within the parameters of a "normal" personality may similarly lead observers to point to a lack of self-control when more severe symptoms develop. All too frequently we hear people say, "Why not just exercise more self-control and not give in to psychotic, depressive, or manic behavior?"

> It is no surprise that the stigma of mental illness has been very strong in Western culture because our society places a high value on self-control, free will, and individual responsibility. It is not difficult to see how these values, coupled with ignorance, have led to the public view of mental illness as a sign of character weakness.

CONTRIBUTORS TO STIGMA

The major factors creating and perpetuating the stigma attached to mental illness are fear, ignorance, and shame.

Fear

Fear is a powerful determinant of stigma. It is often a reflexive reaction when observing behaviors that don't make sense and appear unpredictable. People may be especially fearful of the impulsive or confusing behaviors evidenced during psychosis or severe forms of mania. Despite all the research demonstrating that people with mental illness are actually less prone to violence than others, many people are still fearful because aggressive behavior is erroneously associated with mental disorders. Although 3 percent of mentally ill patients could be categorized as dangerous, television programming, as well as the news media in general, portray those with mental illness as being strongly responsible for a vast number of crimes, including murder.[4]

Feeling fear and anxiety can be a natural reaction to encountering someone with a mood disorder. When you are in the presence of someone with severe depression, you quickly notice the look of hopelessness, helplessness, and despair and feel how all zest for life is gone from that person. These observations can raise fear and anxiety, especially in those who have the slightest propensity for depression. They are reminders of uncomfortable attitudes and emotions that we struggle with to avoid experiencing. Even people who approach life with optimism and passion may experience anxiety when a loved one is severely depressed. They may experience confusion, a lack of understanding, and a sense of helplessness to make things better.

Feeling fear and anxiety can also be a natural reaction in someone who witnesses a person exhibiting extreme mania. The behaviors associated with mania might be especially threatening to people who are concerned about losing control of their own passions and impulses. In a culture that values self-control, the bold, daring, and colorful actions of those with mania may seem outlandish, "over the edge," and overly self-focused.

Ignorance

Ignorance is a major contributing factor to the responses of fear and anxiety. Between lack of knowledge and basic confusion over how to explain someone's behavior, people are likely to become anxious and concoct subjective and irrational explanations for the behavior as a means of easing their own anxiety. This is as true for the observer of such behaviors as it is for the person with bipolar illness displaying the behaviors.

Ignorance also directly contributes to the stigma of mental illness. A lack of knowledge about the causes and treatment of mental illness keeps stigma, and the practices based on stigma, firmly in place. For example, insufficient training or experience may lead a family physician, relative, or friend to minimize the need for further assessment and treatment of an individual suffering bipolar symptoms. Quickness to minimize or deny depression and a tendency to evaluate symptoms of mania as within the norm both reflect and promote the stigma that interferes with an accurate diagnosis.

Lack of knowledge may also foster social isolation of those with mental illness. A lack of knowledge regarding the course of bipolar disorder or its treatment, or the belief that one just needs to exercise greater willpower, intensify the experienced sense of stigma that pressures those afflicted with mental disorders to not seek treatment.

In the late 1960s, the mental health field made an effort to provide more humane treatment for patients with mental illness by transferring many of them back to their communities from state psychiatric hospitals. Community mental health centers (outpatient services, inpatient units, day-care programs, and group homes) were established to provide the necessary continuum of care for patients. With the advent of improved medications and the structure provided by these community mental health centers, it was hoped that patients would experience less isolation, be helped to stabilize, and return to a higher level of functioning.

> *Ignorance directly contributes to the stigma of mental illness. A lack of knowledge about the causes and treatment of mental illness keeps stigma, and the practices based on stigma, firmly in place.*

During these years, it was the philosophy of mental health treatment teams to make every effort not to hospitalize patients experiencing emotional crises. Staff would spend hours, even days, with as many family members as possible to provide structure and help stabilize the patient. Avoidance of using the community inpatient unit was not based on cost efficiency (HMOs were not yet a dominant force in health care), but on the clinical view that hospitalization would have an extremely negative impact on the patient's overall self-esteem. Although well intended, this approach unwittingly communicated a stigma associated with hospitalization. Embedded in the philosophy of the approach was the message that hospitalization equaled failure. When hospital admission was deemed necessary, the patient felt defeated, experiencing admission as lost self-control, failure to measure up to self-expectations and the expectations of others, and letting down one's family and treatment team.

Shame

The experience of shame is at the core of stigma. Shame affects not only the mentally ill, but also those living with the afflicted. Recent studies reflect the notion that the foundation of shame involves the awareness of not living up to one's own code of standards, rules, or norms or those of others.

> The experience of shame is at the core of stigma. Shame affects not only the mentally ill, but also those living with the afflicted.

A component of shame is the negative self-judgment or evaluation that follows awareness of not measuring up to "the code." To the degree that such standards are perceived as important and widely held by others, they more frequently are internalized. Violation of these internalized standards leads to a negative self-assessment. Much of the fear, anxiety, and guilt surrounding mental illness are based on ongoing and pervasive efforts on the part of the afflicted and their loved ones to avoid this painful experience of shame.[5]

Michael Lewis clearly articulates the experience of shame and differentiates it from guilt. Shame is a self-reflective observation that involves an appraisal of one's whole self. In contrast, guilt is a self-reflective emotion by which one identifies a specific action as not measuring up to self-expectations or the standards set by others. While guilt is painful, it is not all encompassing. Guilt often leads to defining an action that can be taken to rectify a situation whereas shame does not. Shame is much more profound; it is experienced as a sense of wanting to disappear, hide, or even die—a total escape.[6]

> *While guilt is painful, it is not all encompassing. Shame is much more profound; it is experienced as a sense of wanting to disappear, hide, or even die—a total escape.*

REFLECTIONS ON SHAME

Kathy Cronkite, who had her own experience with depression, interviewed celebrities and politicians who experienced severe depression or bipolar illness. The following is Cronkite's compilation of how those with mood disorders view shame.

For example, Mike Wallace said he did not experience shame over the prospect of losing his job. Nevertheless, he worried about being fired for depression.[7]

William Styron told Cronkite that he did not experience shame. "You feel shame only when you've done something that you're derelict about," said Styron. "I had enough awareness to know that this was not my fault."[8]

"Jane Doe," a Washington, D.C., professional who did not wish to be identified, reported that shame and related stigma are prevalent in our nation's capital. "People don't have feelings here, and they don't have problems, nor disease, nor depression, nor sadness."[9]

In her conversation with Cronkite, Kitty Dukakis suggested that we often think of people who can't function in society when we look at mental illness. "That's probably one of the reasons that more people don't come forward and get the help they need. I hid it, but other people who are mentally ill can't put up a veil and hide it. The tragedy is that so many people, particularly people in highly visible positions, don't get the help they need because of their concern about what the public will perceive."[10]

Experience of Shame

The four key features that form the experience of shame are:

1. The desire to hide. "Hiding" occurs on many levels. Feeling shame may lead a person to isolate physically from others. People may practice social isolation or withdrawal in an attempt to decrease their vulnerability to their shame and to new shame-provoking experiences. Increased inhibition in all forms of self-expression may be another attempt to avoid potentially shame-provoking experiences. Hiding can also be expressed in ways that involve distracting oneself from the experience of shame by emotional substitution, focusing on other emotions instead of the shame. Through denial and minimization, the person becomes consciously aware only of the anger and/or depression that are consequences of experiencing shame.[11]

2. Feeling intense pain, discomfort, and anger. The pain experienced in shame is very intense. The self-evaluation of not living up to a standard leads one to experience hurt, sadness, and overall shame. Anger can develop as an outgrowth of the discomfort from these negative emotions and may be directed at oneself or toward others as a distraction from experiencing shame.

3. Feeling no good, inadequate, and unworthy. The interplay of the self-devaluation and the experience of pain escalates and in-

Whether in the public eye or not, shame can lead to isolation by those living with bipolar disorder. And when those with this disorder, and those who live with them, ignore, minimize, or deny the seriousness of this illness, they foster such shame. Even statements intended to provide support may further shame and isolation. For example, advice such as, "Just force yourself a little at a time, you can do it," or "Say some positive affirmations when you wake up and before you go to sleep," may provide some measure of support for those with low-level depression. Severely depressed individuals, however, experience these gestures of help as exhortations that

tensifies to the point of producing a feeling of complete worthlessness. Scholars who have studied attribution theory (the area of inquiry that tries to identify to what factors people attribute their successes and failures, self-esteem, and optimism-pessimism) emphasize that depression is related to internalizing blame for negative events.[12] Shame is based on a negative assessment of the whole self and experienced as permanent.[13]

4. The self focuses completely on itself. Objectivity in self-evaluation is lost and confusion prevails when one assesses oneself as being totally inadequate. When we reflect on ourselves, assessing our shortcomings from an intensely negative and "all-encompassing" point of view, self-doubt and anxiety prevail and any action is viewed as futile. This paralyzing quality of shame inhibits one's capacity to think clearly, talk, or act.

When the shame of mental illness is so culturally ingrained and pervasive, leading to a generalized reaction involving the whole person, it is easily understandable why people with bipolar disorder view themselves as "depressive" or "bipolar" rather than as an individual with a mood disorder. The illness becomes the identity, and shame exacerbates depression when one's entire identity is experienced as the illness.

come at a time when they feel powerless to implement such practices. The gestures of help only add to the shame felt as a consequence of failing to measure up to expected standards. However, even though well intended, the mere avoidance of any discussion about the illness, its symptoms or impact, may also further contribute to the stigma of bipolar disorder.

In several of her books, author Susan Sontag explores the meanings that we have come to associate with various illnesses. For example, according to Sontag, we developed a romantic view that those with TB experienced tremendous passion that remained unexpressed. In contrast, she says, "The romanticizing of madness reflects in the most vehement way the contemporary prestige of irrational or rude (spontaneous) behavior (acting-out), of that very passionateness whose repression was once imagined to cause TB, and is now thought to cause cancer."[14]

However, meaning given to illness has changed through the ages. While the former view was that a certain illness corresponds to a specific character, in recent years, we view illness as an expression of the character. As Sontag notes, "It is a product of will. Recovery from a disease depends on the healthy will assuming dictatorial power in order to subsume the rebellious forces of the sick will."[15]

> The tragedy is that so many people, particularly people in highly visible positions, don't get the help they need because of their concern about what the public will perceive.
>
> —KITTY DUKAKIS

This view has serious implications for the promotion of shame. Walk into any bookstore and you'll see many books in the medical, psychology, and self-help sections focused on improving physical or emotional well-being. While many of these offer powerfully constructive ideas, others reflect Sontag's concern: "The romantic idea that the disease expresses the character is invariably extended to assert that the character causes the disease because it has not expressed itself."[16]

This notion promotes shame and perpetuates stigma as it puts the onus of disease on the patient. Sontag states that our culture views illness as a psychological event and encourages people to believe that they unconsciously will it. It is this view of illness that, even in our "enlightened" society, still places stigma on both those who experience mood disorders and on their families. When language implies that the individual is responsible for his or her illness, it reinforces blame, guilt, and shame, and reduces the desire to seek treatment.

RESPONSIBILITY AND STIGMA

Frequently, those who blame victims of mental disorder for their illness suggest that the afflicted are just giving in, being self-indulgent, avoiding responsibility, or being manipulative. Exploring these charges in more detail illuminates their circular reasoning. What might be the motivation of "giving in" to depression or psychosis? If one is self-indulgent, what is the incentive to indulge oneself in feelings of shame, guilt, and even paralysis of thought as experienced in severe depression? What intensely uncomfortable subjective experience makes one feel unable to be responsible or work toward meeting his or her own needs? What intensely negative internal experience leads one to avoid responsibility or to try to manipulate others?

When we focus on the idea of pretense, that the illness is a ruse or a strategy just to get one's needs met, we fail to take notice of the real pain associated with mental illness. In fact, staying with this focus is a way to avoid recognizing pain in others. However, if we acknowledge that someone's pain is real, we also accept the needs and desires of that person. This capacity to understand serves as the foundation for compassion.

Let us consider the evolution of how our attitude toward responsibility influences our view of mental illness. As suggested in the writings of Sontag, we are more likely to blame people for their condition to the degree that we can attribute responsibility to them. Sontag cited one study that found that more stigma is attached to overweight people and to those with AIDS than to people with cancer. The assumption is that individuals can do something about their weight and sexual behavior, but we have no control over developing cancer.

Research that demonstrates the biological and neurochemical etiology of severe depression and bipolar illness encourages the afflicted to feel less responsible for the illness. Both the medical community and advocacy groups emphasize these findings to provide education about appropriate attitudes and treatment and, thereby, reduce stigma. This educational thrust should be supported and applauded.

At the same time, this view may have tremendous implications for establishing guidelines for compassion. Does it indirectly suggest that we develop a hierarchy for compassion? Should we feel more compassion for nonsmokers with cancer than for smokers with the disease? What about people with severe depression whose condition is viewed as chemical in origin; should we have more compassion for them than for those who experience less severe depression? If our focus is on the concept of free will as fundamental to guiding behavior, we are more prone to blaming a victim of depression, especially if we don't believe in the biological or neurobiological basis. When that is the case, we are, in fact, limited in compassion.

Part of the blame, as reflected by the culture of self-help, lies in the way we view the underlying motivations of individual thought, feelings, and action. If we do not identify a biological component, we more readily look for the role individuals play in developing and maintaining their state of depression. To the degree that mental health practitioners have made us aware of competing or unconscious motivations, we can use these motivations as ammunition against those who experience emotional disturbance. But is it really in our control?

> If our focus is on the concept of free will as fundamental to guiding behavior, we are more prone to blaming a victim of depression, especially if we don't believe in the biological or neurobiological basis.

A more discerning and mature adult might say, "If only I had the wisdom then that I have now, I would have made better decisions." That small word "if" makes all the difference. Once depression sets in, the condition takes over and the afflicted individual exhibits symptoms of the disorder: lack of awareness, narrowed vision, and constriction of thought, behavior, and emotions. During periods of extreme depression or mania, the person only minimally experiences choice, if at all. In addition to chemical imbalance, depression can be related to a lack of resilience as a result of genetic factors, cumulative stress, and experienced trauma. Should people with these conditions be the target of anger, either self-directed or derived from others?

"HOW GOOD DO WE HAVE TO BE?"

In his book *How Good Do We Have to Be?*, Harold Kushner discusses how we have raised our standards from "striving to do well" to concentrating on the need for perfection. This is the standard we apply when we stigmatize mental illness. We invariably sow the seeds for depression through unrealistically high self-expectations. These expectations are activated by a society bent on perfection; we seek perfection in our weight, in our appearance, and in all the expectations we have of ourselves and others.[17]

How do Kushner's views apply to the stigma of mental illness? It is our idealization of perfection that keeps us from exercising compassion, not only toward others but toward ourselves as well. If we accept our common humanity and that we are all imperfect beings, compassion will follow. Whether mood disorders are biologically related, stress related, or a result of trauma, we can be accepting.

Lack of compassion, which is both a cause and a result of stigma, has a significant impact on the experience of individuals with mood disorders. Regardless of the etiology of the illness, part of the experience of being depressed is helplessness, hopelessness, and reactions that extend beyond sadness and hurt to despair. Stigma affects the management of depression before, during, and after all stages of the illness. The very thought of saying out loud that you are depressed often leads to fear of what people will think, fear of rejection and/or abandonment, and fears about job security. Those who are depressed may be surrounded by family and friends who support these same fears, either consciously or unconsciously.

The lack of knowledge about mental illness that is associated with stigma can also foster the isolation of the afflicted person. If you are unaware of appropriate treatments for depression, you might engage in self-talk, such as, "I'll let it pass . . . I'll see what happens . . . It'll go away . . . I need to keep my image up." Consequently, untreated depression leads to increased isolation, further reducing one's experience of being effective, having needs met, and feeling connected with others. It also fosters and reflects a loss of compassion for oneself.

To draw a parallel with physical illness, imagine ignoring severe and lingering chest pains, fever, a suspicious and expanding growth, or the onset of blurred vision. Delaying medical treatment can have serious consequences and make the condition more difficult to reverse.

Depression can produce an inability to concentrate that may interfere with work performance. Frequent mistakes lead to interpersonal conflicts and tension, which exacerbate the fears of the afflicted person, and diminishes performance quality. Stigma and shame, already associated with the disorder, are then further exacerbated as the afflicted individual feels less and less effective in his work.

A severe manic episode may also interfere with effective work and overall performance. However, the sense of shame and related stigma may not be experienced until a period of emotional stability when one is more able to reflect on bizarre or inappropriate behaviors.

It is equally important to identify the impact of the mood disorder stigma on friends or family of the afflicted person. This is primarily significant in recognizing how their reactions might influence the seeking or avoidance of treatment. Even when those around us are trying to be compassionate, they may be affected by fear, ignorance, and shame. Sometimes these can stem from a friend or relative not feeling helpful, being fearful of saying or doing the wrong thing, becoming frustrated, feeling anxious about the future, or even experiencing shame or guilt by association.

> *Stigma affects the management of depression before, during, and after all stages of the illness. The very thought of saying out loud that you are depressed often leads to fear of what people will think, fear of rejection and/or abandonment, and fears about job security.*

Fear, ignorance, and shame related to stigma can combine to induce anger and resentment. As mentioned previously, people may even believe that their depressed or manic friend is malingering, being overly self-indulgent, or manipulative. But a severely depressed person is self-focused, not necessarily procrastinating, being overly self-indulgent, or controlling. Nobody wants to remain in the depths of depression.

If manipulation occurs, it is because depressed people are also fearful and feel ashamed. They might be unprepared to exercise self-help due to lack of knowledge. Although some individuals develop an identity around an illness, severe depression is not an experience one fully chooses to maintain. Using illness as a crutch rather than attempting to improve the situation is a sign of fear, anxiety, deficient knowledge, lack of trust, or another block that keeps the person feeling unable to move forward. Regardless of the origin of depression and manic-depression, mental illness deserves compassion, not anger; acceptance, not stigma; understanding, not ignorance and bias; and respect, not devaluation.

> Regardless of the origin of depression and manic-depression, mental illness deserves compassion, not anger; acceptance, not stigma; understanding, not ignorance and bias; and respect, not devaluation.

REDUCING STIGMA: PRACTICING C.A.R.E.

The practices that work most significantly to dispel stigma fall into four specific categories: compassion, advocacy, recognition, and education, which form the acronym C.A.R.E.

Compassion is an essential ingredient in reducing stigma, whether practiced by a person who suffers from bipolar disorder, a friend or relative of someone who is afflicted, or merely an interested bystander. Compassion is not a goal, but a way of being that is part of an ongoing process. When someone is sympathetic to the pain of another, it reduces stigma. When someone expresses sensitivity and respect toward self and others, it challenges fear. When a person is forgiving rather than holding out for perfection, it eliminates stigma.

Compassion demonstrates and fosters connection with oneself and others, challenges isolation, and promotes healing. It involves a fully conscious choice and commitment to this way of being. As an ongoing process, we need to choose compassion on the many occasions that require it. Those who live with people afflicted with bipolar disorder can choose compassion. In contrast, only minimal choice exists for those who are severely depressed or manic because during an acute episode too much is happening for an ill person to handle.

Advocacy is a major activity in reducing stigma. Advocacy may involve the promotion of increased education, the funding of research, the support of legislation, or any of a variety of activities that both directly and indirectly reduce stigma. Through individual efforts or group involvement, advocacy both empowers and is an expression of empowerment. Advocacy helps alleviate stigma by influencing political, social, economic, and medical policies. Advocacy is most strongly epitomized by the work of organizations such as the National Depressive and Manic-Depressive Association (National DMDA) and the National Alliance for Mental Illness (NAMI). Through their active community involvement with politicians, doctors, lawyers, religious leaders, and educators, these groups help reduce stigma. Professional mental health organizations, such as the American Psychiatric Association and the American Psychological Association, also play an effective role in advocating for patients' rights and for the practices and policies that eliminate stigma. Each group provides and generates funding for education and continued research to improve the quality of treatment for bipolar disorder.

Recognition of mood disorders is needed before we can put a "face" on mental illness. It is no surprise that movements to combat stigma associated with illnesses such as bipolar disorder were initiated by those who live with the conditions. Celebrities and noncelebrities alike who publicly address their trauma or illness give bipolar disorder a face. Their courage in going public helps reduce fear and ignorance by reminding everyone of our shared humanity; we feel more connected. Whether we're informed about breast cancer by a well-known actress, bipolar disorder by a noted television news journalist, AIDS by an Olympic gold-medal swimmer, substance abuse by the wife of a United States president, or domestic violence by a relatively unknown man or woman in rural America, sharing helps everyone deal more effectively with life's many challenges. The courage of others enables those who are afflicted with bipolar disorder to feel less isolated in their own struggles.

Education combats stigma and promotes compassion by presenting facts that help to eliminate fear and ignorance. Education is the primary goal of advocacy groups like NAMI and National DMDA—as well as the American Psychiatric Association and the American Psychological Association, both of which provide books, pamphlets, and videotapes on all forms of mood disorders. Each year, the American Psychological Association schedules a day for screening depression at hundreds of sites nationwide. While adults have traditionally been the targeted audience, other programs are being developed to reach out to young people. In a pilot project conducted in a rural area of northern Mississippi, a high school presented a program through discussion, lecture, and contact with those afflicted to help reduce the stigma of mental illness and prevent adolescents from being ridiculed about the disorder. Several months later, when students who had participated in the program were reassessed about their attitudes toward mental illness, they consistently responded with more positive attitudes than those who had not taken part in the program.[18]

> *Celebrities and non-celebrities alike who publicly address their trauma or illness give bipolar disorder a face. Their courage in going public helps reduce fear and ignorance by reminding everyone of our shared humanity.*

Recently, the American Psychological Association initiated the most comprehensive campaign ever to fight the stigma of mental illness among young people.[19] Launched in June 2000, and supported by Tipper Gore as an outgrowth of the White House Conference on Mental Health (1999), this five-year program seeks to transform the public's basic perceptions and attitudes about mental health. Joining with the APA executive director for practice, Dr. Russ Newman, Gore emphasized, "We cannot discriminate just because the illness happens to emanate from the brain, which is a part of the human body, a part of the human condition . . . but apparently we have to educate people about that."

Partners in this effort include the offices of the United States Department of Health and Human Services, the United States Surgeon General's Office, the National Institute of Mental Health, the Office of the Assistant Secretary for Planning and Evaluation, and the Substance Abuse and Mental Health Services Administration. Specific goals include greater access to health care for people with mental disorders, and decreased discrimination for them regarding employment and housing.

Based on a highly successful campaign against youth violence, "Warning Signs," APA, in conjunction with MTV, has developed and begun airing 60-second announcements that urge the audience to "Change your mind about mental health." Viewers are encouraged to call a toll-free number (800-964-0009) or log onto www.NoStigma.org in order to obtain a pamphlet, "Change Your Mind About Mental Health: A Get-Help Guide for Teens and Young Adults." The brochure discusses depression, panic disorders, and eating disorders and presents guidelines for getting help.

SUMMARY

Schools should be the starting point to help combat stigma. Even in the lower grades, teachers can inform children about mental illness at a level commensurate with their intellectual and emotional understanding. These issues need to be addressed, not treated as if they don't exist. Only by openly confronting the subject can we hope to broaden public awareness, understanding, and sensitivity so that society can embrace a higher level of compassion. Since fear of the unknown is the most frightening fear of all, education is our best tool for eliminating stigma.

The combined efforts of the four practices of C.A.R.E.—compassion, advocacy, recognition, and education—offer powerful avenues for expression and empowerment while helping to dissipate stigma by transforming shame to compassion.

CHAPTER 8

Optimism, Hope, and Transcendence

W HAT ROLE DOES optimism play in the life of someone with bipolar illness? If optimism can influence the course of illness, what impact does optimism have leading up to, during, and following a severe depressive or manic episode? Are hope and optimism related? Can a person be inoculated with optimism, just as one receives a vaccine to ward off the flu virus? Is it possible to transcend bipolar illness or, perhaps, develop better coping skills to manage the disorder?

Let us examine these questions and explore their relation to the experiences that are part of bipolar illness.

Optimists Versus Pessimists

In recent years, optimism has become a serious topic of concern for those who study attribution theory, the area of inquiry that tries to identify to what factors people attribute their successes and failures. According to Martin Seligman, one of the more widely recognized writers on this topic, pessimists tend to believe bad events will last a long time, will undermine everything they do, and are their own fault. Optimists view a defeat as a temporary setback and its cause specific to the situation. In addition, optimists tend to believe circumstances, bad luck, or other people caused the event to happen. Confronted by a bad situation, they perceive it as a challenge and try harder.[1]

The Art of Hope

Hope may best be described as a cousin of optimism. Seligman views "the art of hope" as being able to find temporary and specific causes for misfortune. He suggests that "temporary causes limit helplessness in time, and specific causes limit helplessness to the original situation." Another definition of hope is "uncertain pleasure" in anticipation that one's wishes will come to pass. Depression and mania are both conditions that show marked shifts in the ability to experience optimism and hope.

Transcendence

Transcendence involves the ability to move beyond one's current situation. It reflects the concept that people are evolving, dynamic, and shifting beings rather than static creatures. We are not stagnant in our thinking or in our emotions or behavior. This concept places a high value on self-awareness and being able to step outside of ourselves to observe realistically our own life as a moment in transition. Transcendence gives us the power to imagine ourselves in a wide range of potentially different situations.

> Transcendence involves the ability to move beyond one's current situation. It reflects the concept that people are evolving, dynamic, and shifting beings rather than static creatures.

Transcendence is reflected in many ways, sometimes by behaviors that span years, months, or even moments. We can learn from an example related by Bernie Golden of an event that took place several years ago during a vacation he took in Hawaii with friends. His group of six discovered an isolated beach. Within ten minutes after two of them had gone off swimming, the other four heard someone scream for help. At first they thought it was a joke, until they spotted one friend thrashing about in the water. Both swimmers had been caught in a riptide, but only one was in serious trouble. Bernie, a former lifeguard, dashed immediately into the water to rescue his panic-stricken friend. As he helped him to shore, his friend stared dazedly, and Bernie noticed the man's face turning blue. The friends on the beach assisted him as Bernie waded out again to help the second swimmer to shore. That swimmer was calmer, alternating swimming parallel to the shore and lying on his back. He met Bernie halfway out and they returned to shore together.

That evening, the others questioned the more relaxed swimmer about what he'd been thinking during the riptide mishap. He answered that he had instinctively instructed himself to remain calm, that the shore was right there. "Don't panic," he told himself. When in a riptide, one needs to swim with the tide instead of fighting it. He knew to stay parallel to the beach until he was able to move closer to shore.

Though caught in a riptide, Bernie's friend had been able to focus visually and emotionally and maintain thoughts of being safely carried back to shore. A major aspect of transcendence is abstract thinking: being able to project an image of oneself over time toward a positive shift from the current predicament, rather than fixating on one's plight and the initial fear and anxiety that it provokes. Transcendence, therefore, is the ability to orient oneself beyond the immediate limits of any given time and space and to think in terms of "the possible." According to Rollo May, the author of *Existence*, it is this capacity to imagine and look beyond the current situation that we refer to as the basis of human freedom.[2]

A unique characteristic of human beings is the ability to see a vast range of possibilities available to us in any situation, depending on our self-awareness and capacity to run through in our imagination all the different ways we could react to that situation.[3]

OPPOSITE POLES: DEPRESSION AND MANIA

Anyone who has experienced, or observed someone experiencing, severe depression or mania knows that during this intense phase there is self-awareness, but the capacity for objective self-awareness is radically diminished. During the more severe episodes of depression, a person is unable to see possibilities, while during severe mania one is consumed by possibilities. Consequently, one's capacity for self-awareness and self-reflection is not totally absent either before, after, or during certain periods of bipolar illness. The exploration of optimism, hope, and transcendence becomes more relevant when we accept this view of mood disorders and can identify the presence, or absence, of these qualities during the various stages of mood transition. This exploration leads to increased understanding and management of both the depressive and manic experiences.

We might characterize the alternate states of bipolar illness as representing two opposite ends of a continuum. This analogy can easily be understood by listing the specific behaviors, thinking, and subjective experience associated with movement toward each of the opposing ends of the continuum. While the manic state, in its most severe form, encompasses feelings of inflated self-esteem with heightened grandiosity and delusion, an extreme depressive experience is burdened by an overriding sense of inadequacy. Extreme mania is characterized by the experience of unlimited possibilities and potential with absolute disregard for danger or social structure. Depression, in its most severe form, is characterized by negative tunnel vision. Mania focuses on movement toward a future that is optimistic and without bounds; severe depression reflects emotional entombment of the past with no perceived potential for change.

> *During the more severe episodes of depression, a person is unable to see possibilities, while during severe mania one is consumed by possibilities.*

During severe depression, we might experience only pessimism; pessimism can be defined as the absence of hope, constriction by negative thoughts that often don't allow for objective self-awareness and compete with stepping outside of and reflecting on one's experience. In sharp contrast, during severe mania, we experience unrealistic optimism and undaunted hope but, at the same time, are so distracted that the capacity for objective self-awareness and reflection barely exists.

While bipolar disorder is often conceptualized as on a linear continuum, that image does not fully reflect the illness. As Kay Jamison has observed, although manic and depressive symptom patterns clearly have a polar quality, the overlapping, transitional, and fluctuating aspects are enormously important in describing and understanding the illness as a whole.[4]

> *While bipolar disorder is often conceptualized as on a linear continuum, that image does not fully reflect the illness. Although manic and depressive symptom patterns clearly have a polar quality, the overlapping, transitional, and fluctuating aspects are enormously important in describing and understanding the illness as a whole.*

Depression

In *Touched with Fire*, Kay Jamison recounted her personal experience with bipolar illness, which began in high school with a manic period that spanned several months, followed by severe depression. Here, she describes that depression:

"The bottom began to fall out of my life and mind. My thinking . . . was torturous. Nothing made sense . . . all of a sudden, my mind had turned against me. . . . It was incapable of concentrated thought and turned time and again to the subject of death; I was going to die, what difference did it make?"[5]

During this period of despair, Jamison lacked optimism or any sense of hope. She focused on death, decay, and the bleakness and hopelessness she perceived all around her. She emphasized key aspects of depression, including helplessness and hopelessness, and her inability to effect change in her condition. And, what was most debilitating was her despair at the thought that her future held no promise of change whatsoever. While not directly articulated, she referred to overall feelings of inadequacy. And, similarly, though unvoiced, many people in Jamison's severely depressed state experience intense shame.

In the midst of all of this, what was the quality of her self-awareness, her capacity for self-reflection, and her potential for transcendence? Her detailed description of her subjective experience is evidence of her capacity for self-awareness during and after the experience. What was significantly absent during this time, as she herself described so vividly, was the capacity to envision herself as having a different subjective experience, one with greater openness, optimism, and hope. It is the paralysis of not being able to imagine an alternative experience that is the hallmark of intense depression.

In its most severe forms, depression not only involves constriction in thinking and emotions, but may also be reflected in the person's physical demeanor through muscular rigidity, slowness in movement, and diminished fluidity in facial expression.

Those who have studied depression have noted that there is a slightly altered constellation of symptoms at the less severe level. While still characterized by pessimism and a lack of hope, these qualities are less intense at this level of depression. Similarly, during less severe depression, there is often a greater range of potential for realistic observations. Jamison explored this issue in her comprehensive study of manic-depressive illness and temperament. As mentioned previously, Jamison found considerable data suggesting a profound correlation between bipolar disorder and creativity, with the highest creativity occurring during the early, or less severe, episodes of mania. She also found that many of her subjects described the ability to respond creatively and be actively productive during periods of less intense depression.

According to studies presented by Seligman, those individuals who seem mildly pessimistic also appeared more realistic than those on the optimistic end of the spectrum. Thus at the more mild level of pessimism people are able to realistically assess the potential for negative events to occur. This view is further supported by Shelly Taylor, the author of *Positive Illusions*. While Taylor is provocative in her view that positive mental health is, in fact, fostered by positive self-illusions, she also suggests that those who fall into the category of "mild depressive" can be more realistic in overall perceptions.[6]

Though people may be experiencing mild depression, they may be better equipped to be self-aware and evidence transcendence. Not being bound by positive illusions, they are more able to attend to the full range of positive and negative realities of life. At the same time, low-level depression still leaves one with energy that may be channeled through the expression of one's experience. Creative artistry—writing, painting, or composing music—reflects a capacity to translate subjective experience into something different. This clearly involves a forward momentum and active engagement, even if the creative work focuses on pessimism and lack of hope. Artists are able to disengage from the moment long enough to reflect on their experience and translate it into a new form of expression. Their art may be motivated by personal catharsis, but also by the wish to connect with others.

Mild Mania

Further exploration of optimism, hope, and transcendence, and their relationship to bipolar disorder, is informative in terms of both the illness and basic human nature when we delve more deeply into the mild level of mania. Most of us can readily identify with the experiences of this level of mania. However, most people have these experiences only occasionally, whereas for those prone to low-level mania, these episodes are a more constant, pervasive state.

Mild mania (hypomania), marked by a constellation of positive thinking and emotions, can occur at any time, whether the person is engaged in work or leisure. Nancy describes her experience of this state as follows, "At times I've encountered this experience when actively involved in writing, or thinking about writing. Then I am immersed in my thinking, my thoughts flowing one into another, choosing one path to follow, ignoring another, but with a momentum that almost feels self-propelled. The ideas flow with minimal hesitation and inhibition, while I think thoughts and print them with a sense of visceral, emotional, and intellectual excitement. It is with a sense of abandon and sheer joy that I select words to articulate my beliefs, attitudes, and feelings. Momentum increases and words flow easily. During these moments of heightened creativity, I experience little self-doubt and, as the momentum escalates, I feel little self-consciousness. I might literally, for a moment, lose awareness of my surroundings because I'm so totally immersed in work; all sense of time is lost. The experience of complete freedom to be myself enables me to feel 'in control.' Both during and after this time, I may experience an elevated sense of self-esteem because my writing clearly matches and reflects externally my internal experience. Being fully engaged in the here and now with no sense of past or future, the intense joy of the moment is greatly amplified. While engaged in this writing task, several hours may slip away without my even realizing that I have forgotten to eat!

> Most of us can readily identify with the experiences of this level of mania. However, most people have these experiences only occasionally, whereas for those prone to low-level mania, these episodes are a more constant, pervasive state.

"Intense involvement may interfere with patterns of sleep. When I'm engrossed in self-expression, I often find it difficult to disengage long enough to get to bed at a 'respectable' hour. In fact, I don't mind continuing the process in my head for hours on end because this heightened sense of clarity furthers my emotional high, excitement with life, sense of engagement, and overall feeling of worthiness. I may feel driven and, while not fully aware, I seem to experience the strongest sense of optimism and hope at these times."

Intensely pleasurable experiences like Nancy's may fill entire days for those with low-level mania. Kay Jamison also described the positive aspect of her early manic episodes: "My manias, at least in their early and mild forms, were absolutely intoxicating states that gave rise to great personal pleasure, an incomparable flow of thoughts, and a ceaseless energy that allowed the translation of new ideas into papers and projects."[7]

During this phase, hope and optimism abound and are influenced by thinking that for the most part is realistic, but at times can reflect faulty, unsound reasoning. A decrease in self-consciousness and self-awareness occurs as the person becomes totally engaged in both thinking about and enjoying the intense pleasure of the activity. Thus transcendence is part of this experience, reflected in the immersion.

Optimal Experience: In the Flow

What has been described, up to this point, is part of the constellation of experiences of someone who lives with low-level manic intensity. On looking at the list of "symptoms," many people might express eagerness for similar experiences in their own lives.

In recent years, researchers, while not necessarily motivated to shed light on manic-depression, have tried to examine what factors contribute to enhancing the general quality of life. Mihaly Csikszentmihalyi, a leader in this field and the author of *Flow: The Psychology of Optimal Experience*, studied the psychology of optimal experience and identified components of this subjective experience. His specific findings and conclusions are based on a study of hundreds of individual responses. The participants, who came from different economic levels, different cultures, and had different career paths and interests, were asked to describe optimal experience—those moments of deepest joy.

Csikszentmihalyi refers to the optimal experience as "flow": "The state in which people are so involved in an activity that nothing else seems to matter; the experience itself is so enjoyable that people will do it even at great cost, for the sheer sake of doing it; it is something that we make happen, a moment when a person's body or mind is stretched to its limits in a voluntary effort to accomplish something difficult and worthwhile."[8]

The conditions Csikszentmihalyi defined as necessary components for optimal experience seem to parallel certain qualitative aspects of the core experience of people with low-level mania:

- A task that can be completed

- Full concentration on the task at hand

- A clear set of goals

- Immediate feedback

> The conditions defined as necessary components for optimal experience seem to parallel certain qualitative aspects of the core experience of people with low-level mania.

- Acting with a deep, effortless involvement that removes from awareness the worries and frustrations of everyday life

- Enjoyable experience that allows one to exercise a sense of control over one's actions

- Concern for self disappears yet, paradoxically, the sense of self emerges stronger after the flow experience is over

- All sense of duration of time is altered; hours pass by in minutes, and minutes can seem to stretch into hours

As Csikszentmihalyi suggested, "The combination of all these elements cause a sense of deep enjoyment that is so rewarding people feel that expending a great deal of energy is worthwhile simply to be able to feel it."[9]

Such moments of optimal experience encountered while working, strolling through a park, enjoying a good book, engaged in an interesting discussion, or participating in an enjoyable pastime like scuba diving, swimming, or dancing involve deeply felt positive experiences in which one feels completely immersed in the activity of the moment. Much of the experience of low-level mania appears to encompass such optimal experience. Whether we're talking about emotional reactions, thoughts, actions, or visceral reactions, people with low-level mania report experiences that involve aspects of "flow."

Kay Jamison's research into the lives of artists and writers diagnosed as manic is relevant to "flow" and low-level mania. In a review of changes experienced by these artists and writers, she discovered patterns of behavior during periods of intense creativity that provide terms strikingly similar to the major components of flow.

The Downside of Low-Level Mania

If low-level mania were characterized only by positive experiences, there would be no need for a diagnosis. Hope and optimism flourish and provide the impetus for envisioning a widening spectrum of possibilities in one's daily life. Hypomania includes more than the positive qualities that foster optimal experience, however. It can also involve irritability, distractibility, inflated self-esteem, and a decreased need for sleep (perhaps a maximum of three hours or less).

These qualities can interfere with concentration during flow, reduce one's flexible capacity to disengage from the flow experience, and may involve unrealistically positive judgment of the experiences. Similarly, a person may become excessively involved in some pleasurable pursuit; even during periods of low-level mania this has a high potential for painful consequences such as neglecting one's responsibilities or the need for sleep.

> If low-level mania were characterized only by positive experiences, there would be no need for a diagnosis. It includes more than the positive qualities that foster optimal experience, however.

Ellen, 22 years old, was diagnosed as hypomanic. When Bernie first met her, she appeared extremely light and energized in both her tone of voice and in her movements. Ellen wore her hair in a free-flowing style, which she rapidly and repeatedly brushed away from the side of her face. Her makeup was noticeably bright; though not garish, it overly accentuated her cheekbones and intense eyes. Ellen's animated speech was somewhat pressured as she spoke about her career as an executive secretary and her delight in finally deciding to return to school to pursue a graduate degree in English. She chatted nonstop about her love for poetry, plays, and fiction, and recited passages from her favorite works. Ellen appeared affable and personable, was passionate about life, and showed vitality, hope, and optimism.

Kay Jamison wrote of her similar apparently positive state, "Mood in hypomania is usually ebullient, self-confident and often transcendent, but it almost always exists with an irritable underpinning, fluctuating and volatile. I raced about like a crazed weasel, bubbling with plans and enthusiasms, immersed in sports, staying up all night, night after night, out with friends, reading everything that was not nailed down, filling manuscript books with poems and fragments of plays, making expansive, completely unrealistic plans for my future. The world was filled with pleasure and promise; I felt great. Not just great. I felt really great. I felt I could do anything, that no task was too difficult. My mind seemed clear, fabulously focused, and able to make intuitive mathematical leaps that had up to that point entirely eluded me."[10]

> As the symptoms of mania increase in intensity, the overall experience can move in a more negative direction. Optimism and hope continue strong, but are increasingly influenced by less rational thinking.

In Ellen's case, it was only after several meetings with Bernie that she discussed the difficulties she was experiencing. Her troubles were quickness to become irritated, especially when experiencing blocks to her self-expression; escalating impulsiveness; and increasingly unrealistic self-expectations regarding time commitment and the balance of her involvement with her work life, leisure activities, and friends.

For both Jamison and Ellen, optimism and hope were prevalent. Yet as the symptoms of mania increase in intensity, the overall experience can move in a more negative direction. Optimism and hope continue strong, but are increasingly influenced by less rational thinking.

The person can imagine different ways of being, but they are less based in rationality. Self-awareness, as evidenced by the ability to observe patterns in one's thinking, emotions, or actions, diminishes as mania increases.

Extreme Mania

In describing her own experience, Jamison sums up the more intense period of a manic episode: "Almost everything was done to excess; instead of buying one Beethoven symphony, I would buy nine; instead of enrolling in five classes, I would enroll for seven; instead of buying two tickets for a concert I would buy eight or ten. I was working 20 to 30 hours a week in order to pay my way through college, and there was not a margin at all for the expenses I ran up during these times of high enthusiasm. Unfortunately, the pink overdraft notices from my bank always seemed to arrive when I was in the throes of the depressions that inevitably followed my weeks of exaltation."[11]

As mentioned previously, extreme mania encompasses inflated self-esteem with extreme grandiosity and delusion, and the experience of unlimited possibilities and potential with disregard for any real danger or social structure. It focuses on movement toward a future that is unrealistically optimistic and without bounds.

It was this extreme optimism and distorted thinking that propelled Ellen, during one of her most severe attacks of mania, to saunter boldly into the director of admissions office for a graduate program. There, she demanded immediate acceptance into the master's program. She was determined to be admitted despite her being three courses short of completing her undergraduate degree. Ellen had never engaged in any formal application process and, in fact, had never spoken to, nor made an appointment with, the director of the program. She was finally admitted to the hospital following this bizarre episode and related altercations with campus security.

It is a major challenge in manic illness to monitor and modulate the positive attributes and experiences before they escalate and shift toward a destructive outcome. It is the lure of flowlike experiences that takes hold at the onset of a manic episode and maintains a stranglehold against seeking medication, much less observing compliance in taking it.

THE ROLE OF OPTIMISM, HOPE, AND TRANSCENDENCE IN TREATMENT

In Seligman's view, a healthy and rewarding life is greatly influenced by one's level of optimism versus pessimism. Similarly, he focuses on how a person's "explanatory style" may influence his or her placement on the optimism-pessimism scale. According to Seligman, the explanatory style is the manner in which you habitually explain to yourself why events happen.[12] It is that inner voice that offers meaning, makes appraisals, and explains events. As mentioned in an earlier chapter, this internal voice can be so *inner* and so habitual that we are unaware of being engaged in self-dialogue.

To illustrate the explanatory styles of pessimism and optimism, let's consider the example of a screenwriter who fails at his first attempt to sell a script to a movie company. Intense pessimism is reflected in an explanatory style that concludes that he will never sell the script, that he is most likely to fail at other endeavors, and that his failure is based on poor writing skills or, even worse, on his overall inadequacy. An optimistic explanatory style, on the other hand, views the rejection as a single event, without assuming that his other projects are heading for a similar fate. The writer looks for other explanations of rejection, such as lack of budget, timing, and insufficient interest in the subject. He weighs all factors equally, and his focus is outward rather than thinking the fault lies with him.

Optimists are more realistic about externalizing the cause of negative events. The word "realistic" needs emphasizing, as Seligman indicates, because during depressive episodes people frequently exaggerate their personal responsibility for a negative event. Likewise, falsely externalizing the causes is an escape from responsibility. Seligman suggests that some degree of pessimism is healthy, especially when based on a good "reality check." This implies assessing the realities of a situation before taking, or during, an action.

Our behavior is largely the result of modeling and internalizing the styles of people with whom we shared significant relationships during our formative years. For example, a parent may instruct a six-year-old to think optimistically by helping the child understand that a writing mistake is a specific error rather than a sign of the child's general inclination to make mistakes continuously.

Seligman's views have many implications for bipolar illness. Further, he has developed programs based on his theories to help instill optimism and treat various forms of depression. His methods help people recognize and monitor the underlying thoughts that foster an optimistic or pessimistic explanatory style. Once they recognize these underlying thoughts, the program helps them acknowledge the realistic optimistic thoughts and challenge the pessimistic thoughts with more accurate and realistic explanations. For example, people can reduce catastrophizing by identifying specific and temporary causes in contrast to their global and pervasive explanations for negative events. Similarly, they can challenge their quickness to overvalue their contribution to negative events by identifying a variety of realistic external explanations for what caused the event.

> People can reduce catastrophizing by identifying specific and temporary causes in contrast to their global and pervasive explanations for negative events.

Cognitive behavioral psychotherapy incorporates Seligman's ideas about explanatory style (see chapter 5). As with other therapies, more severe forms of depression, especially when connected to manic-depressive illness, require drug therapy before an individual can benefit from his approach to optimism.

Hope, as discussed earlier, involves identifying temporary and specific causes for misfortune. This capacity is one of the major ingredients in an optimistic explanatory style.

Understanding explanatory style can provide new insight into the experience of transcendence as it applies to bipolar illness. Anyone who is severely depressed or manic is unable to be truly transcendent if we focus on the part of transcendence that includes the ability to envision realistic possibilities for oneself. But how do people with bipolar disorder explain, or make sense of, the illness when they are only slightly depressed or manic (before and after an episode)? How does one's explanatory style about one's condition impact the illness?

If we maintain a pessimistic explanatory style about our bipolar illness, this "explanation" can foster depression about the depression. We will feel more depressed, less hopeful, and less optimistic if we think in terms of always being in a permanent state of mania or depression, we overgeneralize all negative aspects of life as related to our illness or core being, or we tend to personalize the cause of the illness (as something we have control over or contribute to). We are then constricted in our sense of potential and more likely to label ourselves manic-depressive, as distinguished from a person *with* manic-depression. This difference, though subtle, has tremendous implications for the way we view our illness and the manner in which we seek and follow an appropriate course of treatment.

> When the larger society communicates negative messages about illness, afflicted individuals are bound to internalize and adopt this thinking as their own. They learn to accept a pessimistic explanation for mental illness, which, in turn, diminishes their capacity to transcend the effect of the illness.

Seligman's concepts regarding depression also help to provide insight into the social impact on bipolar illness. We the afflicted, and those with whom we have significant relationships, are all part of a larger culture that helps to develop our explanatory style. Our society sends very clear messages regarding mental illness, particularly bipolar disorder. It's been a relatively short time since people have begun to view mental disorders more realistically and compassionately. It has been an even shorter period since the public first began to recognize bipolar disorder as a condition of intense mood cycles that can be regulated with medication and are time limited, not permanent.

When the larger society communicates negative messages about illness, afflicted individuals are bound to internalize and adopt this thinking as their own. They learn to accept a pessimistic explanation for mental illness, which, in turn, diminishes their capacity to transcend the effect of the illness.

It is a lifelong challenge for those who live with bipolar illness—an ongoing process of developing and maintaining optimism and hope in the face of all the internal and external factors that *could* convince us otherwise.

ENHANCING OUR CAPACITY FOR TRANSCENDENCE

The essential task in living with bipolar disorder involves a constant struggle to remain alert to the signs that this illness, by its very nature, is constantly working to undermine our capacity to accurately self-judge. Staying alert involves vigilance in developing an explanatory style about our illness that favors realistic optimism and hope. We need to rethink how we explain events, especially the illness itself. It is important to note that in recent years new strategies have been identified to help develop this vigilance and to increase the capacity for meaningful transcendence.

Researchers have devoted much attention to finding new ways of managing emotions, since our emotions impact our behavior and attitudes. Psychologist and author Daniel Goleman has written extensively about the concept of "emotional intelligence." This form of intelligence refers to our abilities to motivate ourselves by persisting in the face of frustrations, to control our impulses and delay gratification, to regulate our moods, and to empathize and to hope. Goleman notes, "When emotions are too muted, they create dullness and distance; when out of control, too extreme and persistent, they become pathological, as in immobilizing depression, overwhelming anxiety, raging anger, manic agitation."[13]

According to Goleman, emotional intelligence is a "meta-ability," a constellation of abilities that allows us to oversee, to monitor, to make use of, to create balance with, to marshal, and to integrate our emotions. It is a weakened capacity to think realistically and implement emotional intelligence during the extreme states of depression that leaves us unable to move forward.

While Goleman has identified thirteen groups of abilities that compose emotional intelligence, four are most relevant for coping with bipolar illness. These are described below.

> It is a weakened capacity to think realistically and implement emotional intelligence during the extreme states of depression that leaves us unable to move forward.

Self-Awareness   Self-awareness involves the ability to reflect on oneself and recognize one's feelings, having a vocabulary for labeling those feelings, and understanding the relationships between thoughts, feelings, and reactions. Self-awareness is a key issue for anyone with mood disorders. The ability to recognize and differentiate emotions, as well as the intensity of each emotion, allows you to identify markers on the path of escalating mania or spiraling depression. Similarly, self-awareness focuses on being able to differentiate thoughts from feelings and recognize the interaction between and amongst them. This type of awareness does not require obsessive, paralyzing, self-conscious self-absorption. It can, especially in the beginning, be fostered by the use of daily journaling, as often suggested in treatment and in self-help books. External feedback, in the context of psychotherapy or support groups, is essential to identify patterns of thinking and associated emotions more clearly.

Personal Decision Making   Personal decision making includes the abilities to explore your actions, recognize and anticipate their consequences, and be aware when emotions or thoughts serve as the basis for your decisions. Personal decision making calls for pushing a pause button on the forward movement of your intended action. The pause allows for self-reflection, clarification of actions and potential outcomes, understanding if thoughts or emotions are ruling the action, and recognizing what is in your best interest.

Insight   Insight involves the abilities to identify patterns in your thoughts, emotions, and actions and to recognize patterns in others. The capacity to have insight regarding your own emotions, thoughts, and actions makes you more sensitive to recognize the complexity of their interplay in the actions of others.

Managing Feelings   Managing feelings is based on several abilities that include the capacities to identify automatic thoughts that are self-critical, recognize the complex interaction of emotions (for example, anger is so often a secondary to hurt, feeling devalued, or rejection), and to manage negative emotions such as fear, anxiety, anger, and sadness. The ability to manage feelings, especially intense and negative ones, increases your tolerance for frustration. Recognizing, identifying, and challenging negative self-dialogue contribute to your ability to manage your feelings.

We live in a world that is highly complex and continually changing, in a society in which we experience constant challenge to learn new skills. It is important in this environment to regard emotional growth and development as an ongoing process—it takes time, patience, and commitment. Likewise, it is an ongoing process to develop one's emotional intelligence.

> *Recognizing, identifying, and challenging negative self-dialogue contribute to your ability to manage your feelings.*

By describing the experience of bipolar illness, we have more clearly identified the challenges that must be addressed in managing and coping with this illness. In addition to identifying the challenges faced by people with bipolar disorder, this analysis offers insight into the form and timing of treatment. These concerns can best be addressed by viewing a summary of our exploration of the ebb and flow of optimism, hope, and transcendence associated with bipolar illness.

As reflected in table 4, severe depression brings with it intense pessimism, hopelessness, and diminished ability to step outside of one's experience and objectively observe that experience. This reduced capacity to observe one's thinking and emotions interferes with the ability to be optimistic, experience hope, and envision transcendence beyond one's current situation. During this phase, those with bipolar illness are very much in need of external support and involvement.

Table 4. The Ebb and Flow of Optimism, Hope, and Transcendence in Bipolar Illness

	Severe Depression	Mild Depression	Stable Phase	Mild Mania	Severe Mania
Optimism/ Pessimism	Extremely pessimistic	Pessimistic	Typical for person	Highly optimistic	Unrealistically optimistic
Hope	Hopeless	Some	Typical for person	Hopeful	Unrealistically hopeful
Openness to transcendence	Closed	Somewhat	Typical for person	Extreme	Unrealistic in extreme
Realistic thinking	Impaired	Increased	Typical for person	Mixed	Impaired
Objective self-reflection	Impaired	Increased	Typical for person	Mixed	Impaired

In this phase, treatment focuses predominantly on strengthening and restorative approaches rather than proactive approaches. This severe, paralyzing form of depression requires medical attention. The use of medication therapy and maximizing contact with others, especially those who can be supportive, empathic, and realistic, are two forms of needed support during this phase. Those with severe depression can be helped at this time by psychotherapy that focuses on providing support and education rather than on the learning of completely new skills for managing emotions and thinking.

The primary focus of treatment during this phase is to prevent the symptoms from worsening and promote the slightest increase in the patient's capacity for optimism, hope, and transcendence. Another major focus should be on helping the person establish and maintain emotional connection, with loved ones as well as with others who have had similar experiences with depression. In this phase of the illness, the patient is faced with concerns about trust and issues about illness and accepting help in general. So while an individual with severe depression may be least open to socialize, even with others who may have had similar experiences and can provide support, it is at this time that such support is most necessary.

> This reduced capacity to observe one's thinking and emotions interferes with the ability to be optimistic, experience hope, and envision transcendence beyond one's current situation.

Similarly, strategies that are most helpful at this time are those that help reduce constriction in thinking. This is facilitated by assisting the afflicted in trying to revisit a part of themselves, by accessing memories of times when they experienced more optimism, hope, and transcendence. While severely depressed, they may not be receptive to learning new strategies of thinking, but should be encouraged to rely on realistic self-talk that has previously been employed to challenge pessimistic, devaluing, and negative thinking. Even reviewing journals, written at a time when they experienced feeling optimism, hope, and transcendence, can help challenge the severe depressive thinking of this phase. It is important to remember, however, that depression drains energy and concentration, so even these strategies may not be consistently well received.

During mild depression, people have an increased capacity for self-awareness and an ability to reflect on thoughts and emotions and the patterns they form in influencing the current life experience. In this phase, they can engage more in strengthening and restorative approaches and more constructively channel their energy to manage the depression.

In this phase, depressed individuals may be most open to participation in psychotherapy, either individual or group, or in self-help groups. They may also be most open to learning strategies for fostering constructive optimistic thinking, skills for challenging distortions in thinking as practiced in cognitive therapy, and emotional skills in the context of therapy. Although the depression is less severe, the afflicted still very much need the support of others, especially as such assistance offers sound reality checks to their negative views of themselves and life in general. In fact, they may be most open to treatment during this phase because they are motivated to alleviate the discomfort of the depression.

During the stable phase, people experience optimism, hope, and transcendence in ways that are typical for their particular personality and least influenced by the deteriorating impact of extreme depression or mania. During this period, they may be most able to learn strategies of coping with their illness that are proactive rather than reactive and restorative in focus. It should be emphasized that during mild depression, the stable phase, and mild mania, people may be most available to channel their energies and concentration in developing skills to cope with depression and mania. As the depression is alleviated, as a greater sense of well-being emerges, or as mild mania intensifies, motivation for treatment may begin to diminish.

During the stable phase, people should be most encouraged to step back and observe their illness. This is the ideal time to develop new ways of thinking that become a natural part of their repertoire, so they can respond more favorably to future life challenges that might otherwise influence their movement toward depression and mania. Whether keeping journals, maintaining logs of their experience, making use of bibliotherapy (incorporating the use of self-help books in treatment), or therapy techniques focused on pausing to self-reflect, this is a time for increasing the skills of self-monitoring thoughts, emotions, and behavior.

As people become more strongly influenced by mania, even during the mild phase, the increase of energy, optimism, and experiences that approach the flow experience can decrease the motivation to take time to reflect and learn new skills.

During severe mania, people are least motivated to make use of treatment and least able to recognize the need for it. Unfortunately, conflicts with others, including the law, during this period often lead to a referral to treatment.

It should be emphasized that major change can still occur during the extreme phases of both mania and depression. Specifically, the individual may acknowledge the need for medication and other treatment. It is during the other phases, however, that the most significant changes can take place in terms of learning how to understand and manage bipolar illness.

> As depression is alleviated, as a greater sense of well-being emerges, or as mild mania intensifies, motivation for treatment may begin to diminish.

SUMMARY

We have explored how optimism, hope, and transcendence impact and are impacted by bipolar disorder. Complete management of bipolar disorder requires transcendence—a working together of emotion and intellect in order to move forward. We need to be able to shift our thinking beyond a knee-jerk response and regulate our emotions. This requires close monitoring. To the degree that we can learn to anticipate and recognize the subtle and not-so-subtle signs of shifting moods, and to the degree that we can learn new skills to modulate these moods, it is possible to constructively channel our energies toward a life that yields greater joy, fulfillment, and productivity.

Certainly, drug therapy is essential to help manage severe depression and mania. However, the work of Csikszentmihalyi, Seligman, and Goleman provides specific ways of observing our emotions and thinking. This is not passive observation of uncontrollable prevailing moods and thoughts, but, rather, an active engagement in feeling and living. With these abilities, we can directly observe and alter our emotional life in a positive way. These skills are essential ingredients for optimism, hope, and transcendence; for coping with emotional trauma; and for the management of manic-depression.

The advent of new medications and the increased awareness of the psychological and emotional needs of those afflicted with bipolar disorder (and those who live with them) make it possible for the afflicted to learn to value themselves, maintain rich lives, and develop new strategies to reduce the negative and devastating effects of their illness.

CHAPTER 9

The Spirit of Self-Help

I have suffered, but I know that without the suffering, the
growth I have achieved would have been impossible.

—*VIKTOR E. FRANKL*

IF VIKTOR FRANKL could survive a Nazi concentration camp
and rise above the horror of it all, those of us with bipolar disorder
ought to be able to find ways of managing our own situation. But
where do we find a safe haven? Frankl found peace at Auschwitz when
he looked up and saw the clear blue sky. Something in him allowed
him to be open to beauty despite his surroundings of war and hate. At
that moment, Frankl was no longer a prisoner; his body was held captive, but his soul remained free.

Our biological needs must be met to maintain good physical and
mental health, but a true and lasting happiness also rests on our ability to reach beyond the basics. Frankl was stripped of everything except life itself, but he credited his survival with never having lost
hope. "Only those who were oriented toward the future, toward a
goal in the future, toward a meaning to fulfill in the future, were
likely to survive," said Frankl.[1]

In search of the meaning of life, those of us with bipolar disorder must first acknowledge that our primary goal should be to improve our quality of life. Since our very survival depends on our well-being, to compromise health jeopardizes life. The basic ingredients of life are sleep, food, love, sex, and money. First, we must force ourselves to get adequate rest. During periods of low-mania it is easy to go for long periods of time with minimum sleep since those afflicted tend to function on adrenaline. But, lack of sleep affects our body's immune system, making us more vulnerable to disease. Second, exercise builds healthy bodies and helps keep us "balanced" by diffusing excess energy and warding off bouts of the blues. Third, diminished appetite and compulsive eating habits are also traits of manic-depression, and a concerted effort must be made to concentrate on a healthy diet. Finally, paying close attention to the needs of one's partner brings people closer together. Perhaps our most basic need of all is to love and be loved. Happiness cannot be purchased, and nothing compares with peace of mind.

When taking a proactive approach to bipolar illness by monitoring health, we can focus on pursuing meaningful goals.

SETTING A GOAL

We can start by setting a realistic goal, a unifying purpose for the things we do in our everyday lives. A "realistic" goal means one you can reach. If your goal is unrealistically high, you might feel threatened, insecure, or unqualified to achieve it. If you under-challenge yourself, the goal won't serve its purpose of providing meaning and orienting you to the future.

Mini-goals are the stepping stones that lead you to your final target. Setting mini-goals allows you to experience success and learn to manage frustration while in pursuit of your main objective. If you succeed in meeting all necessary requirements to accomplish that final goal, then you will have gained the necessary tools and confidence to reach even further.

With every passing decade our society becomes more advanced technologically. To survive, and thrive, in such a fast-moving culture we must continue to grow as individuals. Rather than cling to old patterns of behavior, we can find untold fulfillment and joy by being adaptable and open to learning fresh skills. However, those of us who live with bipolar disorder also have the additional burden of maintaining emotional balance while pursuing our goals. The following list will provide guidance:

1. Establish your basic needs. As individuals, we vary greatly in our basic needs and in our ability to achieve those needs. For some, mere survival is paramount and overrides anything else, which by comparison represents unaffordable luxury. Basic survival is dependent on having a roof over our heads, food, clothing, and companionship. To succeed in life, we must monitor our health. When our bodies are sleep deprived or lack proper nutrition, the result can be eyestrain, headaches, and general malaise and fatigue.

2. Expand your horizon. After the basics of food and shelter have been met, you can begin to expand your horizon by turning your attention and your energy to other aspects of life. An individual who has achieved personal security has the ability to be more open and available to family, friends, and the community. For some, life becomes focused around job concerns, educating children, and doing their best to provide for their family's happiness and well-being. Each of us is challenged in different ways, but our best moments often occur when our mind or body is stretched to the limits. Enjoyment and fulfillment can be attained by forward movement, a sense of novelty and accomplishment that may have seemed unimaginable before. Some experiences may not be pleasurable at the moment, but appreciation comes later when we look back. The result of such encounters leads to personal growth.

3. Achieve a healthy and safe interdependence. Some people develop strength and self-confidence by clinging first to family for security, then branching out independently. Some women, for example, become more independent after marriage because of the security they derive from the relationship with their spouse. A healthy and safe interdependence allows both spouses to become more independent.

Bonding and accepting intimacy is important since we, by our very nature as human beings, are social creatures. Intimacy is letting oneself feel close, open, honest, and trusting of another human being. The ideal relationship becomes a mutually bonding one, connecting our life with others—parent, teacher, sibling, spouse, lover, or friend—in a mutually beneficial way. Since in a healthy relationship no one dominates over the wishes of another, such a partnership yields mutual respect, trust, and love.

4. Set limits. People who have achieved a high level of independence have learned to prioritize goals and set limits. People who fail to set limits and are controlled by success are vulnerable to becoming obsessed.

Watch Out for Obsession

In working to meet whatever goals we have set, those of us with bipolar disorder need to be wary of becoming obsessed by achieving those goals, since obsessiveness is a characteristic of our illness. Obsessiveness can have both positive and negative outcomes. Being obsessive—spending too much time being extremely organized and focused—certainly speeds the mastery of skills in any new area of growth. In excess, obsessiveness can lead to a successful career at the cost of intimacy or full participation in family life. Too frequently, the end result is a wrecked marriage and estranged children. People in this situation may be left wondering if their success was worth it.

If your goal is so exciting that you become fixated on it, the price you pay to attain that goal may be too high. Anyone can fall victim to this trap when limits have not been set. People in a state of fixation can focus nearly all of their attention and energy on themselves. Others become absorbed in a compelling project or cause to the exclusion of relationships with family and friends (self-indulgence and inattentiveness to others are traits of mania/hypomania). This is what happened to Nancy.

"When I first dove in as a Soviet Jewry activist, I had no special skills or training for this job, other than the desire to be involved and to help," said Nancy. "I enjoyed the camaraderie of belonging to a group, I found a mentor, and little by little I learned. Our organization had a goal and collectively we were determined to accomplish our mission. Not until later did my preoccupation with Yuri become so intense that I became an unsuspecting victim. Had I first established limits, I would not have been entrapped.

"Yet it was the mania in me that supplied me with fuel—the energy and strength I needed to accomplish things that might otherwise have seemed impossible, or off-limits! The mania gave me the courage to telephone important political figures.

"Since every manic episode is followed by depression, when you are high there is no place to go but down. The more manicky the episode, the greater the plunge.

"It was during that plunge that I irrationally reached for a bottle of aspirin and swallowed an overdose of pills," said Nancy. "I felt, at that moment, as if I had lost my balance and had plummeted to the bottom of the earth from the peak of Mount Everest. Everything around me appeared to be going up in smoke, and life was being snuffed out."

During the Cold War era of the former Soviet Union, Nancy was offered an opportunity to become politically involved with a national movement to help rescue Soviet Jews from their persecuted state. What first began as curiosity and concern led to a deep commitment and, ultimately, a serious destructive obsession. Nancy began to lose her way after traveling to the Soviet Union and meeting Yuri, the former Russian scientist and political prisoner. Back at home she was catapulted into spearheading his rescue on a worldwide basis. Nancy's main mission and reason for being became Yuri's emancipation. Involved in international affairs and interacting with prominent public figures, Nancy's glamorous and exciting activities were far beyond anything she had imagined herself doing.

"I found it exciting and terrifying, and I could not concentrate on other things."

Nancy's commitment to Yuri's rescue turned into an obsession. Tension soon mounted. Nancy started taking risks that imperiled not only her personal security but her family's. What had started as a noble cause to save another human being turned into a larger-than-life crusade that nearly cost Nancy her sanity.

"I gambled with my marriage and jeopardized the welfare of my children," said Nancy. "I was not always home for them, or was home but unavailable. Other 'needs' took precedence. Nevertheless, I could not stop nor alter my path. I was obsessed with my mission. I wouldn't permit anyone or anything to stand in my way before I had reached my objective."

When Yuri was liberated and at last permitted to emigrate, Nancy found herself without the cause that she had focused her entire being on for five years. Nancy's personal life was in an upheaval, as she and her family were growing desperately apart. She had risen from dilettante to savior, but failed to prepare herself for the "real" world following Yuri's emancipation.

After losing all sense of perspective and control, Nancy eventually found herself on a one-way path going nowhere but down. As a chronic obsessive-compulsive, she was looking for trouble and found it. Nancy's fixation ended with a major depressive episode and a failed attempt at suicide in 1994 when she swallowed an overdose of aspirin. This irrational episode was a desperate cry for help.

INGREDIENTS FOR A FULL, HAPPY, AND BALANCED LIFE

Well-integrated people don't fall into the trap of obsession, but are able to achieve their goals while observing healthy limits. They understand the concept of a truly meaningful life and can succeed without jeopardizing that meaning.

Let us return to the basic ingredients of life, our primary needs: sleep, food, love, sex, and money. If we consider these needs as something greater than mere human sustenance, we can accept the philosophy that the body is capable of many forms of enjoyment, a promising factor in the meaning of life, without going overboard by being obsessive. This is how, and when, those of us who live with bipolar disorder, find ourselves in trouble. We can all learn to find, and to appreciate, beauty in every aspect of life if we follow the guidelines below.

The Importance of Sleep

"Just five more minutes," pleads the child who is glued to the television set and doesn't want to go to bed. But five minutes is never enough, nor is any amount of time ever enough for a bipolar patient who is determined to finish a project.

Just as we need food and water, adequate rest is also necessary for a properly functioning body. This is especially true of people with bipolar disorder.

Nancy may intellectually understand her need for sleep, but she still struggles with the issue: "It is difficult for me to put down a good book that I am reading, let alone put aside a consuming writing project. This is the mania in me! My head refuses to listen to the cries of my body when it screams out for sleep." When Nancy stays up to work and doesn't sleep, she invariably suffers the next day. She feels sluggish, irritable, and suffers from eyestrain after staring at the computer screen all night.

The Importance of Exercise

While exercise is important for everyone, it is critical for people with bipolar disorder. Not only does exercise help to create balance by diffusing the excess energy that is symptomatic of mania, but exercise is equally effective in helping ward off bouts of the blues.

Low-impact exercises such as swimming and walking are less stressful on the body than some of the more rigorous forms of exercise. Eastern body training methods, such as yoga, help to cultivate the mastery of deep relaxation techniques that improve flexibility, soothe the body, and clear the mind. Other Eastern disciplines include judo, jujitsu, kung fu, karate, tae kwon do, aikido, and t'ai chi.

The Importance of a Healthy Diet

Since diminished appetite and compulsive eating habits are traits of manic-depression, those afflicted with bipolar disorder need to make a concerted effort to follow a healthy diet regime.

Allocating sufficient time to eat may not always be possible or practical. While nutritionists point to breakfast as the most important meal of the day, it is frequently rushed because everyone is in a hurry. Men and women rush off to work, and children hurry out to catch their school bus; a continental breakfast (coffee/tea/milk, juice, and toast) too often becomes standard fare. Unfortunately, lunch is frequently eaten on the run, too (if at all). That leaves dinner supplying the bulk of daily nutritional needs. If you are bipolar, your chemical balance is exacerbated by faulty eating habits. By skipping meals, indulging in fast foods, and too frequently pigging out on junk, people with bipolar are more dramatically at risk than others in terms of compromising health and diminishing the overall quality of life.

Dr. Artemis P. Simopoulos, a renowned expert on nutrition, believes that a moderate amount of fat in our daily diet is essential for both mental and physical well-being. In her book *The Omega Plan* (coauthored with Jo Robinson), we learn how the right fats increase our chances of living a long, "lean," and healthy life.

"Fat," states Dr. Simopoulos, "is the raw material for hormonelike substances that virtually influence every function in your body, from your blood pressure to your sensitivity to pain. Your brain is composed primarily of fat, including the neurons that transmit electrical messages; if you don't eat enough of the right types of fats, you are depriving your brain of a critical nutrient and risk falling prey to depression and other mental disorders."[2]

What is the right type of fat? What is the wrong type? Studies have shown that the most harmful fat is saturated fat. Found in meat, dairy products, and some tropical oils, saturated fat increases the risk of coronary artery disease, diabetes, and obesity. Another harmful fat is trans fatty acid. These acids are manmade molecules produced during hydrogenation (e.g., the production of vegetable oil). Simopoulos has demonstrated that an earlier theory, which prompted the switch from butter to margarine, was a bad idea.

Beneficial fats include olive oil and canola oil, which reduce the risk of certain metabolic disorders while protecting the body's cardiovascular system. Essential fatty acids (EFAs) are necessary for normal growth and development and help guard against depression. Two researchers from the National Institutes of Health, Joseph Hibbeln and Norman Salem, found that people who consume a large amount of fish have a low rate of depression. For example, in Japan, Taiwan, and Hong Kong, fish consumption is high and the depression rate is low. If our diet does not contain EFAs, we become deficient in these important fats. Omega-6 fatty acids are most abundant in vegetable oils such as corn, safflower, cottonseed, and sunflower. Omega-3 fatty acids are primarily found in seafood, green leafy vegetables, canola oil, and walnuts. An imbalance of EFAs is linked with a long list of serious conditions, including depression.[3]

The Need for Relationships

We tend to seek out partners who complement us and help us create balance. "In our family," said Nancy, "my husband is the more pragmatic of the two of us. His mathematical mind is quick to focus and he thinks in terms of the bottom line. I, on the other hand, am a detail person and prefer to elaborate. Were it not for my husband's curtailment, I might ramble forever. As an accountant, he is also more practical in financial matters; I'm less conservative.

"As a person who lives with bipolar disorder, I also add spark. Being compulsive, I am driven to complete projects, whether they are personally oriented or ones benefiting both of us. My husband's complaint: if he wakes up in the middle of the night to go to the bathroom, the bed is made by the time he returns. A slight exaggeration, but you get the point!"

Attentiveness to the signals of one's mate tend to bring people closer together; so do shared experiences, raising children, the melding of families, mutual friends, and common goals. But, when people with bipolar disorder are focused inwardly they miss these important signals. A general malaise may develop, and partners may drift apart and form new relationships.

If sex is the most powerful yearning known to humans, it yet pales in intensity when compared with our most basic of all emotional needs—to love and be loved. Love brings peace, harmony, and fulfillment. Since self-indulgence and inattentiveness to others are traits of bipolar illness, those of us who suffer from the disorder must be particularly mindful of the welfare of our loved ones. During periods of heightened mania, we are also more prone to episodes of flirtatiousness and promiscuity. Sex outside of marriage can be addictive and depleting. The dangers are obvious and everybody ultimately gets hurt—spouses, children, parents, and friends alike.

The Joy of Sex

The depth we feel from a sustained relationship can more than compensate for transitory romance. No honeymoon lasts forever; a healthy marriage depends on substance for its long-term survival. Don't bow to temptation when heightened sexuality becomes a problem. Force yourself to think ahead instead of focusing on some immediate sense of gratification. Remember: the cost of your transgression may be too high.

Can Money Buy Happiness?

Success in our society is often equated with how much money a person earns. But, money does not equal happiness. We cannot purchase happiness, although spending sprees are symptomatic of bipolar illness. Money may improve our standard of living, but it cannot replace what is missing in our life if we are struggling with internal discontent. Our most profound need is peace of mind.

SELF-MONITORING

Self-monitoring is an essential self-help strategy for taking a proactive approach to bipolar illness. Ongoing attention to one's stress level and change of moods is a major component of self-monitoring. Stress has a particular impact on people with bipolar disorder. For example, stress more profoundly impacts the onset of the initial depressive episode than subsequent ones. The body chemistry is thrown off balance, thereby blocking one's natural ability to respond appropriately to environmental conditions. Stressful events such as loss or separation can create fear, anxiety, and depression.

How vulnerable are you to stress? Have you ever taken a stress test? Are you vigilant about watching for early symptoms of depression or mania? What are your warning signals? Dr. Susan Musikanth, a psychologist from Cape Town, South Africa, and author of *Stress Matters* and *Depression Matters*, developed the questionnaires that follow to measure stress level and depression. The manic/hypomanic inventory was adapted from Mary Ellen Copeland's *Living Without Depression and Manic Depression*. You can use these questionnaires as tools to monitor your levels of stress, depression, and mania.

> *Self-monitoring is an essential self-help strategy for taking a proactive approach to bipolar illness. Ongoing attention to one's stress level and change of moods is a major component of self-monitoring.*

Stress Questionnaire

Answer the following questions to establish your level of stress. Choose one statement that best describes your response to each question.[4]

1. Your partner's or colleague's behavior upsets you.
   Do you:
   a) explode?
   b) feel angry, but suppress it?
   c) feel upset, but do not get angry?
   d) cry?
   e) none of the above

2. You have a huge pile of work to get through in one morning. Do you:
   a) work very hard and complete the lot?
   b) leave the work and look for other ways to pass the time?
   c) complete what is within your capability?
   d) prioritize the load and complete only the important tasks?
   e) ask someone to help you?

3. A friend makes some unkind remarks about you in conversation with someone else. You happen to overhear.
   Do you:
   a) interrupt the conversation and tell the person exactly what you think of them?
   b) walk straight past and forget about the incident?
   c) walk straight past, but start thinking about revenge?
   d) walk straight past and think about the person?

4. You are stuck in heavy traffic. Do you:
   a) honk?
   b) try to take another route to avoid the congestion?

   c) switch on the radio or cassette?

   d) sit back and try to relax?

   e) sit back and feel angry?

   f) do some work?

   g) you do not have a car so you would not be in a position to make these choices

5. When you play a sport, do you play to win?

   a) always

   b) most of the time

   c) sometimes

   d) never; you play for enjoyment

6. When you play a game with children, do you deliberately let them win?

   a) never

   b) sometimes

   c) most of the time

   d) always

7. A deadline is looming, but you are not satisfied with the work you have done. Do you:

   a) work on it all hours to ensure perfection?

   b) panic because you think you will miss the deadline?

   c) do your best in the time available without worrying about it?

8. Someone tidies up your house/office and never puts things where you left them. Do you:

   a) mark the position of everything and ask the person to put your things in the places you have indicated?

   b) move everything back into place once the person has left?

   c) leave most things as they are—the occasional change does not bother you?

9. A close friend asks you for your opinion about a room that has just been decorated. You think it's terrible. Do you:
   a) admit it?
   b) say otherwise?
   c) only discuss the aspects that you like?
   d) offer suggestions on how to make it better?

10. When you do something, do you:
    a) always try to produce something perfect?
    b) do your best and not worry about achieving perfection?
    c) think that everything you do is perfect?

11. Your family complains that you spend too little time with them because of work. Do you:
    a) worry, but feel that you have no control over the situation?
    b) take work home so that you can be with them?
    c) take on more work?
    d) find that your family has never complained?
    e) reorganize your work so that you can be with them more?

12. How would you describe an ideal evening?
    a) a large and swinging party
    b) doing something with your partner that you both enjoy
    c) escaping the rat race by yourself
    d) dinner with a small group of friends
    e) a family evening doing things that you all enjoy
    f) working

13. Which of the following do you do?
    a) bite your nails
    b) feel constantly tired

c) feel breathless without having been physically active

d) drum your fingers

e) sweat for no apparent reason

f) fidget

g) gesticulate

h) none of the above

14. Which of the following do you suffer from?

a) headaches

b) muscle tension

c) constipation

d) diarrhea

e) loss of appetite

f) increase in appetite

g) none of the above

15. Have you experienced one or more of the following in the last four weeks?

a) crying or wanting to cry

b) difficulty in concentration

c) forgetting what you were going to say next

d) irritation over trivialities

e) difficulty in making decisions

f) wanting to scream

g) feeling that you have no one with whom you can really discuss things

h) feeling that you are jumping from task to task without really completing anything

i) none of the above

16. Have you experienced any of the following during the last year?

a) a serious illness (your own or someone close to you)

b) family problems

c) financial problems

d) none of the above

17. How many cigarettes do you smoke a day?
    a) 0
    b) 1–10
    c) 11–20
    d) 21 or more

18. How much alcohol do you consume in a day?
    a) none
    b) 1–2 drinks
    c) 3–5 drinks
    d) 6 or more drinks

19. How many cups of coffee (not including decaffeinated) do you drink a day?
    a) none
    b) 1–2 cups
    c) 3–5 cups
    d) 6 or more cups

20. How old are you?
    a) 18 or under
    b) 19–25
    c) 26–39
    d) 40–65
    e) over 65

21. You have a very important appointment at 9:30 in the morning. Do you:
    a) have a sleepless night worrying about it?
    b) sleep very well and wake up reasonably relaxed, but thinking about the appointment?
    c) sleep well and wake up looking forward to the appointment?

22. Someone close to you has died. Naturally, you are very upset. Do you:

a) grieve because no one can fill that terrible gap?
b) grieve because life is so unfair?
c) accept what has happened and try to get on with your life?

23. You have gotten into trouble over a problem. Do you:
    a) assess the situation on your own and try to find another solution?
    b) discuss the problem with your partner or close friend and try to work something out together?
    c) deny that there is a problem in the hope that it will go away?
    d) worry about it, but make no attempt to try and solve it?

24. When did you last smile?
    a) today
    b) yesterday
    c) last week
    d) can't remember

25. When did you last compliment or praise someone in your family or at work?
    a) today
    b) yesterday
    c) last week
    d) can't remember

Scoring

Add up your score for each question.

1. a=0	b=0	c=3	d=0	e=1		
2. a=1	b=0	c=1	d=3	e=2		
3. a=0	b=3	c=0	d=1			
4. a=0	b=0	c=2	d=3	e=0	f=2	g=1
5. a=0	b=1	c=2	d=3			

	a	b	c	d	e	f	g
6.	a=0	b=1	c=2	d=3			
7.	a=0	b=0	c=3				
8.	a=0	b=0	c=3				
9.	a=0	b=0	c=3	d=1			
10.	a=0	b=3	c=0				
11.	a=0	b=0	c=0	d=0	e=3		
12.	a=1	b=3	c=0	d=1	e=2	f=0	
13.	a=0	b=0	c=0	d=0	e=0	f=0	g=0
	h=1						
14.	a=0	b=0	c=0	d=0	e=0	f=0	g=1
15.	a=0	b=0	c=0	d=0	e=0	f=0	g=0
	h=0	i=1					
16.	a=0	b=0	c=0	d=2			
17.	a=3	b=1	c=0	d=0			
18.	a=3	b=2	c=1	d=0			
19.	a=3	b=2	c=1	d=0			
20.	a=3	b=0	c=1	d=2	e=3		
21.	a=0	b=1	c=3				
22.	a=0	b=0	c=3				
23.	a=2	b=3	c=0	d=0			
24.	a=3	b=2	c=1	d=0			
25.	a=3	b=2	c=1	d=0			

Score

51–68: Your stress level is low. You show very few signs of stress. You are not a workaholic. You thus show Type B behavior and generally cope very well with stress.

33–50: Your stress level is moderate. You show some stress. You are not a workaholic, but there is some tendency toward it. You therefore show mild Type A behavior and generally do not cope well with stress.

16–32: Your stress level is high. You show many signs of stress. It is likely that you are a workaholic. You thus display Type A behavior and do not handle stress very well.

0–15: Your stress level is very high. You show a great deal of stress. You are a workaholic. You display extreme Type A behavior and your ability to deal with stress is very poor.

Depression Inventory

This assessment tool can help you measure the level of your depression, or determine that you are depression free.[5]

Mood

0	I do not feel sad
1	I feel blue or sad
2a	I feel blue or sad all the time and I can't snap out of it
2b	I am so sad or unhappy that it is very painful
3	I am so sad or unhappy that I can't stand it

Pessimism

0	I am not particularly pessimistic or discouraged about the future
1	I feel discouraged about the future
2a	I feel that I have nothing to look forward to
2b	I feel that I won't ever get over my troubles
3	I feel that the future is hopeless and that things can not improve

Sense of failure

0	I do not feel like a failure
1	I feel I have failed more than the average person has
2a	I feel that I have accomplished very little that is worthwhile or that means anything
2b	As I look back on my life, all I can see is a lot of failure
3	I feel I am a complete failure as a person (parent, husband, wife, etc.)

Lack of satisfaction

0   I am not particularly dissatisfied

1   I feel bored most of the time

2a   I don't enjoy things the way I used to

2b   I don't get satisfaction out of anything anymore

3   I am dissatisfied with everything

Guilty feelings

0   I don't feel particularly guilty

1   I feel bad or unworthy a good part of the time

2a   I feel quite guilty

2b   I feel bad or unworthy practically all the time now

3   I feel as though I am very bad or worthless

Sense of punishment

0   I don't feel I am being punished

1   I have a feeling that something bad may happen to me

2a   I feel I am being punished or will be punished

2b   I feel I deserve to be punished

3   I want to be punished

Self-hate

0   I don't feel disappointed in myself

1   I am disappointed in myself

2a   I don't like myself

2b   I am disgusted with myself

3   I hate myself

Self-accusations

0   I don't feel that I am worse than anybody else

1   I am very critical of myself for my weaknesses or mistakes

2a   I blame myself for everything that goes wrong

2b   I feel that I have many bad faults

Self-punitive wishes

0   I don't have any thoughts of harming myself
1   I have thoughts of harming myself, but I would not carry them out
2a   I feel that I would be better off dead
2b   I have definite plans about committing suicide
2c   I feel that my family would be better off if I were dead
3   I would kill myself if I could

Crying spells

0   I don't cry any more than usual
1   I cry now more than I used to
2a   I cry all the time now; I can't stop
3   I used to be able to cry, but now I can't cry at all even though I want to

Irritability

0   I am no more irritated now than I ever am
1   I get annoyed or irritated more easily than I used to
2   I feel irritated all the time
3   I don't get irritated at all at the things that used to irritate me

Social withdrawal

0   I have not lost interest in other people
1   I am less interested in other people now than I used to be
2   I have lost most of my interest in other people and have little feeling for them
3   I have lost all my interest in other people and don't care about them at all

Indecisiveness

0	I make decisions about as well as ever
1	I am less sure of myself now and try to put off making decisions
2	I can't make decisions anymore without help
3	I can't make any decisions at all anymore

Body image

0	I don't feel I look any worse than I used to
1	I am worried that I am looking old or unattractive
2	I feel that there are permanent changes in my appearance and they make me look unattractive
3	I feel that I am ugly or repulsive looking

Work inhibition

0	I can work as well as before
1a	It takes extra effort to get started at doing something
1b	I don't work as well as I used to
2	I have to push myself very hard to do anything
3	I can't do any more work at all

Sleep disturbance

0	I sleep as well as usual
1	I wake up more tired in the morning than I used to
2	I wake up 1 to 2 hours earlier than usual and find it hard to get back to sleep
3	I wake up early every day and can't get more than 5 hours of sleep

Fatigue

0	I don't get any more tired than usual
1	I get tired more easily than I used to
2	I get tired from doing anything
3	I get too tired to do anything

Loss of appetite

    0   My appetite is no worse than usual

    1   My appetite is not as good as it used to be

    2   My appetite is much worse now

    3   I have no appetite at all anymore

Weight loss

    0   I haven't lost much weight, if any, recently

    1   I have lost more than 4 pounds recently

    2   I have lost more than 10 pounds recently

    3   I have lost more than 15 pounds recently

Somatic preoccupation

    0   I am no more concerned about my health than usual

    1   I am concerned about aches and pains, an upset stomach, constipation, or other unpleasant feelings in my body

    2   I am so concerned with how I feel or what I feel that it's hard to think of much else

    3   I am completely absorbed in what I feel

Loss of libido

    0   I have not noticed any recent change in my interest in sex

    1   I am less interested in sex than I used to be

    2   I am much less interested in sex now

    3   I have lost interest in sex completely

Scoring

Add together the numbers you circled. Your total score indicates your depth of depression.

0–9: none   **26–35:** moderate to severe

10–18: mild   **36 and above:** severe

19–25: moderate

Manic/Hypomanic Inventory

This tool can help you assess your susceptibility to manic or hypomanic episodes by monitoring your symptoms. You need to learn what your own early warning signals are and be vigilant about watching for them. Put a check mark next to each symptom that applies to you.[6]

- ☐ insomnia or diminished need for sleep
- ☐ surges of energy and restlessness
- ☐ euphoria
- ☐ flight of ideas
- ☐ excessive planning
- ☐ disorganization
- ☐ inappropriate anger
- ☐ excessive spending
- ☐ diminished appetite or compulsive eating
- ☐ false superiority and grandiosity
- ☐ obsessiveness
- ☐ overambitiousness
- ☐ oversensitivity
- ☐ assuming too much responsibility
- ☐ nervousness and excitability
- ☐ inability to concentrate
- ☐ irritability and outbursts of temper
- ☐ out-of-body sensations
- ☐ others appear "slow"

☐ hyperactivity

☐ incessant chattering

☐ excessive telephoning

☐ self-indulgence and inattentiveness to others

☐ heightened sexuality, flirtatiousness, and promiscuity

Use this list as a reminder of your personal vulnerabilities so you can more effectively monitor the first signs of trouble.

TAKE CHARGE OF YOUR LIFE

It wasn't until I realized that it was up to me to get my moods under control, that there was no magic cure, that I began to turn the corner on the road to wellness.

—MARY ELLEN COPELAND

To begin taking charge of your life, it helps to keep a personal calendar (obtainable through National DMDA; see the appendix, "Resources for Information"). In this way, you can participate in your own treatment by monitoring your mood elevations and depressions. This provides you an opportunity to work collaboratively with your doctor, enabling him or her to regulate your medication more closely. The sample page in figure 9.1 is from Nancy's personal calendar.

Support of Family and Friends

Take a proactive role by informing family members and friends to be prepared for possible warning signals. They can encourage you to stick with treatment. If you become ill, an informed relative or friend will not become offended by mistaking some hasty remark about their "alleged" intrusiveness as a sign of rejection, but will see it as a sign of your illness.

Day of the Week	Medicines I Took (List medicines)	Side Effects (How the medicine made me feel)	Symptoms (How I feel on a scale of 0 to 10 0—most depressed 5—normal 10—most manic)	Activities/ Sleep/Major Life Events (Include "homework" for psychotherapy)	Appointment Schedule
Monday, January 2	None	None	2—depressed Low energy. Irritable. Inability to concentrate.	Slept poorly.	
Tuesday, January 3	One pill at 8 A.M.	None	3—improved mood	Slept better. Forced myself to concentrate on work. Took a walk.	
Wednesday, January 4	One pill at 8 A.M.	None	6—feeling better	Good day at work. Made a list of good things about myself.	Dr. Miller 1:00 p.m.

Figure 9.1—Sample Personal Calendar

During periods of relative calm, it may be helpful to discuss strategy with a loved one to avoid any future problems should another attack occur.

Any threat of suicide must be taken *very seriously*. If the situation becomes desperate, friends and relatives should be alerted that any suicide attempt is a cry for help and to phone the doctor, a hospital emergency room, or 911.

When you're in the recovery stage, advise friends and relatives not to push or be overprotective. They need to understand that you will get well at your own pace, and you need to be treated as normally as possible.

Empowerment

In the spirit of self-help, empowerment is a key factor in achieving the necessary strength and confidence to help yourself. Empowerment is self-assurance, assertiveness, and not being afraid to say no. To feel empowered, you must be able to acknowledge your inner strengths and feel worthy, thereby appreciating your inner self. When you attain self-confidence, you will succeed in gaining the respect, and the attention, of others.

> Empowerment is self-assurance, assertiveness, and not being afraid to say no. To feel empowered, you must be able to acknowledge your inner strengths and feel worthy, thereby appreciating your inner self.

Becoming empowered is a process and cannot be quickly achieved. Like anything else, it takes practice. A piano player does not become a concert pianist overnight, nor is there a magic pill to make us feel empowered. We must, instead, take action. Success can only be attained in a step-by-step process. The following steps are suggested:

1. Develop an adequate support system. A nurturing and healthy interrelationship with another person will offer you that safe haven from which you can grow and develop.

2. Learn problem-solving skills, time management and stress management, and get assertiveness training. Self-help books, such as this one, can offer suggestions and guidance. You can further develop problem-solving skills by attending psychological education workshops (see the appendix, "Resources for Information").

3. Take control of yourself. The actual process of taking control involves great strength, self-determination, and complete self-discipline. It's tough! But keep in mind that anything worthwhile is worth striving for, and this goal has the potential to transform your life.

Authors Ada Kahn and Sheila Kimmel offer suggestions of how to enhance your quality of life through self-empowerment and improved self-esteem. Their method is based on finding ways to eliminate "squashers" (elements that hold you back) while establishing "boosters" (factors that help raise your self-esteem and give you strength).[7]

Emotional baggage—unresolved past issues—is the root cause of many squashers as well as low self-esteem. By confronting negative issues head-on, it is possible to overcome many problems. These issues may have plagued us for years, undermining our self-esteem and making us feel small. Eliminating our "squashers" will reduce stress, pave the way to self-assertiveness, and help us recognize untapped talents and potential ability. Kahn and Kimmel's "Booster Questionnaire" (see sidebar) will help you become more aware of your own strengths and overcome your squashers. You may want to refer to this list on a regular basis to remind yourself of your personal strengths, your accomplishments, and personal pride.

Increase Your Self-Awareness

Swiss psychiatrist/psychologist Carl Jung (1875–1961) was a follower of Sigmund Freud before breaking away to establish his own school of thought: analytical psychology. Jung emphasized the dynamic forces within the individual. Rejecting Freud's focus on sexuality, he believed that the will to survive is more compelling than sexual drive. Jung focused on current problems, rather than childhood conflicts, and developed a theory based on the unconscious mind. "Man is an enigma to himself," said Jung. He concluded that the key to peace of mind is self-knowledge. "An individual, willing to fulfill the demands of rigorous self-examination and self-knowledge . . . will discover important truths about himself."[8]

For many people with bipolar disorder, the turning point in their life comes when they understand their situation, accept responsibility for their actions, and are willing to work hard to change their lives. Finally, they see the light. Although the task ahead may be painfully difficult, simply understanding the problem makes it easier to bear.

"My first confrontation with the need to make radical life changes hit me right after I had plunged into a deep depression following the break with Yuri," said Nancy. "At that critical moment, I felt loveless, friendless, and completely lost, without a career or even a job to fall back on. I turned to my therapist for help."

The challenge of altering one's course in life, after recovering from shock, may ultimately become the motivating force that rewards one with pleasure. In refocusing on something new and different, the change itself can be exciting and stimulating.

Guidelines to Help You Get Well and Stay Well

Mary Ellen Copeland suffered recurring episodes of deep depression, followed by occasional mania, from early childhood until finally seeking medical and psychiatric help as an adult. She went on to become a scholar, teacher, lecturer, and author. Copeland lives with manic-depression, but after conquering her illness she wrote a book to help others get well and stay well. The following guidelines are excerpted from her book and summarize many of the topics we've discussed in this chapter:[9]

1. Believe in yourself! Recognize yourself as a unique and valuable individual, then work at improving your self-esteem.

"Booster" Questionnaire

My strengths are

_____

_____

_____

The aspects of my personality I like best are

_____

_____

_____

I am proud of

_____

_____

_____

What I appreciate about me is

_____

_____

_____

The physical features I like best about myself are

_____

_____

_____

My accomplishments are

_____

_____

_____

Ways in which I take care of myself are

_____

_____

_____

Risks I have taken with successful outcomes are

_____

_____

_____

The personality qualities that make me likable are

_____

_____

_____

What others have told me they admire about me are

_____

_____

_____

Difficult life situations I have lived through, handled, and survived are

_____

_____

_____

When I feel powerful I can

_____

_____

_____

2. Create a network of support, people you care about and can trust to be around when you need them most. These may include family, friends, neighbors, health-care professionals, or members of a support group.

3. Eliminate physical causes of mood disorders:
   - allergies
   - diabetes
   - reactions to prescription drugs or over-the-counter medications
   - drug or alcohol abuse
   - PMS (premenstrual syndrome) or menopause
   - sexual dysfunction
   - thyroid imbalance
   - viral infections
   - vitamin and mineral deficiencies

4. Get a complete physical and neurological examination, starting with your medical history.

5. Discuss the cost factor with your health-care providers (they're in a position to help direct you to affordable programs). Check covered medical services as well as limitations on coverage and its requirements. You can also call the American Medical Association (AMA).

6. Set realistic goals.

7. Stick to a regular exercise program, eat a diet consisting of fresh, natural foods grown without chemicals, and get proper rest.

8. Look for comfortable living space—affordable; easy maintenance; close to community services, family, friends, or other support members.

9. Make time for pleasurable pursuits.

10. Adopt a pet or spend time with someone else's. Pets are healing, reduce stress, and offer unconditional love.

11. Enjoy your career! If your job is not interesting or stimulating, is too far from home, or you don't like your coworkers, change it. Remember, we all have choices. A new job may be your next goal.

12. Get rid of negative influences in your life—people, places, or situations. Anything that causes you stress, anxiety, or depression should be eliminated.

13. Empower yourself! Learn to assume positive action on your own behalf, and take charge of every aspect of your recovery.

IDENTIFYING AND ASSESSING THE REWARDS OF A JOB

You are beginning to take charge of your life by developing a sense of inner awareness. When you begin to feel empowered, take time to evaluate your job. Are you satisfied with your working conditions? Since a large portion of our waking hours is spent at work, every effort should be made to ensure that this part of your daily life is rewarding. If you enjoy what you're doing, you won't feel dissatisfied and bored. For sufferers of bipolar illness, boredom can be a contributing factor to a depressive episode. It frequently leads to anxiety, restlessness, irritability, and anguish. If you remain anchored at a place where you are unhappy, you may feel trapped. Unhappiness and discouragement exacerbate mood disorders.

A positive mental attitude is energizing and helps to encourage you to make whatever adjustments are necessary to improve working conditions. This, in turn, will increase your job satisfaction while simultaneously boosting your self-image and helping you avoid any sense of failure.

When properly challenged, you will not feel bogged down by tedious, repetitive routines that are common to every industry. Although few careers match the responsibility and challenges bestowed on scientists and surgeons, even they can eventually grow tired of their work.

To feel satisfied and fulfilled in your chosen work, it is important to feel appreciated and recognized for your skills. Kahn and Kimmel refer to this as "jobpower." To test jobpower, they developed the Jobpower Scale[10] (see sidebar).

If the Jobpower Scale reveals that you are not finding your job satisfying, you may want to consider looking for other employment.

The sad reality is that job motivation is low in the United States and many people find themselves daydreaming. They might wish they were somewhere else, anywhere else, as long as that "other" place was some distance from work. At the end of the day they return home fatigued and irritable. If you are bipolar and feel trapped in your job, you need to remedy your situation immediately.

How Can You Improve the Job You Have?

If your work environment is uncomfortable but you like what you do, you might be able to remedy the situation by improving your relations with coworkers and bosses. If you want to stay at your job, but find it monotonous at times, look for ways to add variety to your basic job description. Break that routine!

Identify what needs your job satisfies. Not all needs can be met in any one position. You might experience a "lack of fit" when certain needs are satisfied while others are not. Think through whether you can alter your job description to meet more of your needs, or more fully meet some of your needs. Decide if some of your needs can best be satisfied elsewhere. For example, you may work in a position that meets your needs for a good income, social connection, and challenge, but that does not allow you the opportunity for enough creativity. You may decide to maintain the job and seek other outlets for your creativity. Or, you may pursue classes in your area of interest so, with perseverance, you can gain an income from your area of creativity.

If, in the end, nothing you have tried improves your working conditions to your satisfaction, it might be time to look for other employment. A fresh start may be just the thing you need to revitalize your life. Boredom on the job can create major depressions—don't let this

The Jobpower Scale

	Yes	No
Are you satisfied with your job?	☐	☐
Do you feel professionally fulfilled?	☐	☐
Do you feel that you are using your talents and skills?	☐	☐
Are you appreciated at work and recognized for your accomplishments?	☐	☐
Are you in a field you like?	☐	☐
Do others respect you at your job?	☐	☐
Do you feel competent to do the work you do?	☐	☐
Are you paid according to your ability?	☐	☐
Are you getting promotions you deserve?	☐	☐
Are you happy going to work most of the time?	☐	☐
Are you willing to go the "extra mile" to help others in your workplace?	☐	☐
Can you appreciate others' successes at work?	☐	☐
Are you able to speak up to your boss and coworkers?	☐	☐
Are you really interested in the work you do?	☐	☐

The following four questions apply to women only:

	Yes	No
Do you feel you have equality with men at your workplace?	☐	☐
Is your salary comparable to men's for the same job?	☐	☐
Do you get the advancements that men get?	☐	☐
Do men respect you for your professionalism?	☐	☐

If you answered no to more than 5 or 6 of the above questions, your present job may be a poor match for your skills and you may feel trapped.

happen to you. Perhaps a lateral change might be all that's necessary (same type of position, but in a new location), or you may be ready for a career change. Keep your options open.

CHOOSING YOUR OWN DESTINY

The privilege to choose your own destiny and take control of your life offers unconditional freedom. But attainment of this freedom requires a big investment, perseverance, and self-discipline. If you live with bipolar disorder it is of paramount importance not only to self-monitor, but to strictly self-discipline. The prerequisite for this freedom is a positive mental attitude. If you are prepared to meet all the demands of a long and difficult journey, the rewards can be great. It is possible to achieve mastery over your life, and with that comes peace and personal fulfillment.

Your feelings act like a barometer, an internal warning system that is trying to tell you something. Pay attention to those feelings, don't push them away. Accept that a problem exists, think about it, analyze it, and learn from it. If your primary goal is happiness and inner peace, you need to eliminate the obstacles. What is really important? What are your priorities in life? Is it possible that some of your choices may actually have been in conflict with your initial goals?

Know thyself, and listen to your feelings. The little feeling person inside you is saying, "You matter. You deserve to be heard, and I care to listen."

—JOHN GRAY

Stop! Beware of the warning signals, and, do not be afraid. Find some quiet time and space to clear your mind of all extraneous, distracting and self-defeating thoughts. Listen to what your feelings are telling you, or trying to tell you, and heed their warnings. Trust your own intuitions. If you schedule time each day for quiet thought, follow through by sticking to your schedule; it will help you remain "on track."

Krishnamurti described freedom as the ability to see, cast doubt, question everything, and then act on one's feelings and convictions. Those who learn to take action for themselves rather than be dependent on others will find enjoyment and heightened self-esteem in having discarded former strings of bondage in exchange for freedom.[11]

Independent people are far better equipped for life than those who are dependent on others. But, not all dependency is unhealthy. A healthy independence involves knowing when to allow for a healthy dependence, that is, interdependence.

In times of crisis, independent thinkers rely on their own strengths and instincts before going into action. They process, study in detail, and then evaluate every piece of information on possible options. If they choose not to act alone, thinking people can elect to solicit others as team players.

Teammates can learn to work together toward a mutually accepted goal. Independent people know how to ask for help, without being influenced into blindly following someone else. We are bound to make mistakes as we learn to live in this new, healthier way, but this is a learning process that we all must go through.

EXPECT THE UNEXPECTED

What do you do when your best-laid plans are suddenly turned upside down by some unforeseen misfortune? You have prepared for everything—except, of course, the unexpected! A person may feel comfortable and content, both at home and at work, until something happens to upset that delicate balance—sudden illness, problems at work, the loss of one's job, even, perhaps, a forced move out-of-town. A sudden twist of fate—one that seems to jeopardize our very security and well-being—can plunge even the strongest person into despair or a temporary state of imbalance. What then? When "certainty" turns to "uncertainty," how do we cope?

Being creatures of habit, it is human nature to fall back into old patterns of behavior. Some of these old habits may be self-destructive; this does *not* mean to imply that your efforts to take control of and manage your life have failed. Just be prepared to face obstacles. Learn to "let go" when something is beyond reach. Unrealistic expectations are universal, but get past it!

Acknowledge and accept that not everything in life is controllable. Things don't always happen the way we want them to, nor will people always respond favorably to us. Being able to shift gears and move forward in a new direction when confronted by such obstacles is something each of us must learn in order to lead a healthy, well-balanced life.

The ability to make sense out of chaos and rebound quickly is a skill that must be learned. Many individuals who have faced challenging problems have ended up not only surviving, but also thriving. When you have succeeded in developing the necessary skills to help you manage and take control of your life, then you will be ready to appreciate the beauty that life has to offer. Try living in "the moment."

> Being able to shift gears and move forward in a new direction when confronted by such obstacles is something each of us must learn in order to lead a healthy, well-balanced life.

SUMMARY

The best, most comprehensive, and sure way to beat manic-depression is by adhering to the following prescription: psychotherapy, drug therapy, and self-therapy (self-help). No quick cure is available, nor will a pill make the symptoms go away. Bipolar disorder has both biological and psychological roots, and it is a daily struggle to combat the attacks of mania and depression.

Life is an endless series of challenges, but those who become conquerors are true champions. Be honest with yourself and in your relationships. Accept the fact that all people are human and possess human failings. As with any other human weakness, living with bipolar disorder is not easy. Nevertheless, our case studies have illustrated that people with this disorder can, and do, lead very full lives.

You can restore balance to your life, and with balance comes peace. Those who have survived the pitfalls of bipolar illness have discovered health and happiness waiting at the other end. But the ability to get well and stay well is up to each individual. Remember this motto: *The difficult we do immediately, but the impossible takes a little longer.*

CHAPTER 10

A Special Concern
Childhood/Adolescent
Bipolar Illness

WHAT IS IT like to parent a child who has bipolar disorder? The challenge of this undertaking presents one of the most difficult relationships between parent and child.

In preparation for this chapter, we contacted parents who are members of the Child and Adolescent Bipolar Foundation (CABF). We asked them about their experiences and what they most want others to know about living with children and adolescents with bipolar disorder. A common response was, "Our children can be normal and safe when stable." The following examples highlight other responses from the parents.

• **Bipolar illness can manifest at extremely young ages.** "We've been dealing with Steve's illness since he turned one year old. He was such a calm, easygoing infant that we can actually tell you the exact day everything changed with him. Just three days before his first birthday, Steve woke up agitated. When his moods intensified and then continued our family doctor explained our son's behavior by saying that Steve was going through the "terrible twos" even though he was just a year old.

"Each day with him was worse than the day before. Constant irritability, extreme violence, rage, sensitivity to stimuli—touching, lights, sound, everything set him off. He was even affected by tightly fitting clothes, socks with bumps . . . bright lights, loud noises. He was always sensitive to taste and smell. When he was only three years old, the doctor began to suspect he might have bipolar disorder, and by age four we had tried various holistic and behavioral methods. Steve has been on virtually every medication and combination thereof!"

- **Health-care professionals: Please, listen to what we say.**

"Kevin was such a happy baby his first year," said his mother, "but after 14 months, he became very clingy and sad. He couldn't handle changes in routine. In preschool he couldn't focus, he couldn't stay in his seat, and he was very distractible. Kindergarten was more of the same, and by first grade he was on Ritalin. By fifth grade he seemed very unhappy and often cried, but the doctor assured us that our son was not depressed.

"The following year Kevin began to ask questions about what would happen if he were to kill himself. That's when he finally was diagnosed with depression and was started on antidepressants. One year later, in the seventh grade, he experienced his first manic episode and was hospitalized. At that time, we were informed of his bipolar disorder condition and the doctor put him on a combination of Depakote [mood stabilizer] and Zyprexa [antipsychotic/anticonvulsant, originally approved for schizophrenia]."

- **Insurance companies: Please cover this illness like any other medical illness.**

"Brian cried constantly as an infant. He was bothered by hair combing, washing, or touching his head, face washing, and even some unexpected touch. At age two, Brian was aggressive toward his brother and parents. He cursed as a child, showed his genitals, and destroyed property. In school he has been disruptive in the classroom—acting out, deliberately knocking over his desk, and doing anything and everything for attention. At home he is equally uncontrollable—he runs around on the roof, hits his brother with a bat, and has daily rages."

EARLY-ONSET BIPOLAR DISORDER

Imagine waking up and finding your child extremely unmanageable and vastly different from the day before. He may be rageful, have tantrums for hours on end, be impulsive, aggressive to himself and others, and express irritability in his interactions. You become increasingly perplexed as you observe your child's behavior.

You blame yourself, you blame him, and you may even blame your spouse. With each of these reactions, you feel guilt and shame. As parents, you may find yourselves increasingly at odds as the two of you try to cope. A sense of helplessness and frustration often results when a child develops early-onset bipolar disorder.

> As parents, you may find yourselves increasingly at odds as the two of you try to cope. A sense of helplessness and frustration often results when a child develops early-onset bipolar disorder.

You may find your neighbor less friendly, perhaps telling her children not to associate with yours. Perhaps they have observed him, or they may even have been the target of his aggressive behavior. Your neighbor's children don't need to be told to withdraw from him. They instinctively do so.

Early diagnosis is essential for optimal treatment of bipolar disorder, and yet mood disorders in children and adolescents represent one of the most underdiagnosed categories of mental illness. This is especially problematic since bipolar disorder in childhood greatly interferes with a child's capacity to develop a solid foundation of

Message from the Parents

The following are what the parents we interviewed most want others to know about living with children and adolescents with bipolar disorder:

Our children can be normal and safe when stable.

Bipolar illness can manifest at extremely young ages.

When possible, health care professionals should ask the child's history without the child present so he doesn't hear a list of negative behaviors. He already knows!

Don't tell your kids to stay away from mine. He's not contagious.

skills essential for meeting the increasingly complex challenges of maturity.

Since 20 to 30 percent of adult bipolar patients report having had their first episode prior to age 20, early diagnosis is particularly important.[1] Despite these realities, doctors rarely identified bipolar disorder in children (and slightly less rarely in adolescents) until the 1980s.

While some parents may first seek help for a toddler or young child, most parents involved in the Child and Adolescent Bipolar Foundation report that symptoms were either present from birth or developed suddenly during adolescence.[2]

Symptoms of Bipolar Disorder in Children and Adolescents

The symptoms of mood disorders in children and adolescents are expressed somewhat differently than in adults. For example, while a child's depressed mood may at times mirror the depressed emotion,

Health care professionals: Please, listen to what we say. Do not blame us! Have compassion and understanding for us. We need more doctors who specialize in this disorder.

Insurance companies: Please cover this illness like any other medical illness. No more discrimination on mental-health care. My son deserves treatment without our worrying about using more than our "20 days a year" coverage!

It takes a multimodal approach to effect positive change and achieve some stability. Parents are the child's number-one advocate. Listen to them. There is hope for stability.

Please continue to educate others about this illness.

withdrawal, helplessness, and hopelessness characteristic of adult depression, both the mania and depression of bipolar disorder in children are more frequently expressed by behavioral symptoms.

Extreme Irritability and Emotional Lability

Extreme irritability and emotional lability (changeability) are hallmark signs of depression and mania in childhood. Intense irritability may lead to severe tantrums, characterized by their intensity and prolonged duration. Many young children have tantrums that last 20 to 30 minutes and occur occasionally beyond early childhood. In contrast, some children with bipolar illness, as in the case of Brian, cry for several hours during infancy, require little sleep, and evidence a general level of physical excitement and activity well beyond that of the normal infant.

The child with bipolar illness can engage in tantrums for hours without showing signs of reduced intensity. Also symptomatic of bipolar illness are tantrums that seem to abate for several hours only to be resumed again, and for extended periods of time, either that same day or during a consecutive period of days.

Intense Rage

Children and adolescents with bipolar disorder can exhibit intense rage that is expressed both verbally and physically toward peers, parents, siblings, teachers, and even themselves. They may be precocious in the profanity they use to express their rage. Such anger may seem totally unexpected and with no identifiable precipitant. The quickness to act aggressively further reflects the extremely impulsive quality of their thoughts and actions.

Hyperactivity

A lack of impulse control is further demonstrated by the extreme hyperactivity of children and adolescents with bipolar illness. Whereas the average child may have periods of great physical energy, the child or adolescent with bipolar disorder has periods of energy that are out of control and lacking in structure and direction.

> Children and adolescents with bipolar disorder can exhibit intense rage that is expressed both verbally and physically toward peers, parents, siblings, teachers, and even themselves.

The average child may jump from couch to floor while proudly proclaiming, "I'm Superman." He may do this a few times, but the hyperactive child may repeat it 20 times. The child with bipolar disorder may take it to an extreme and jump from the top of a staircase or even the roof. Such behavior may stem from his activity level, coupled with a sense of grandiosity that may impel risk-taking or underlie genuine suicidal ideation.

Sleep Disturbances

Mania in childhood may be demonstrated by a variety of behaviors. Normal children and adolescents can experience sleep difficulties, but the manic child may be too preoccupied at bedtime to sleep. Instead of sleeping, the child may play with toys, rearrange furniture, work on several craft projects simultaneously, move about his bedroom, or rove around the house.

A child may complete many projects and leave others undone, but the manic adolescent with greater freedom than his younger counterpart might experiment with drugs, party through the night, and drive recklessly by speeding while intoxicated.[3]

Miscalculated Life-Threatening Risks

The older manic adolescent or adult may be prone to fast driving or excessive purchasing, but the manic child can endanger his life by miscalculating the potential risk that the average "risk-taking" child or adolescent would not encounter. An example of this is physical challenge involving jumps, leaps, or balancing acts that stretch beyond what is considered a reasonably calculated risk.

Overestimation of Ability

Risk-taking behavior may, in part, be driven by the influence of grandiose thinking. Such thinking may also lead to stealing without any sense of wrongdoing, dictating to adults (teachers, parents, and others) on how things should really be, or obtaining poor grades with little or no sense of possible consequences. Similarly, an adolescent may express strong convictions of his great achievements in sports or music, when in fact he lacks the skills for such achievement. Children may exhibit pressured speech and describe racing thoughts.

Precociousness

Some children and adolescents with bipolar disorder are very precocious in language skills and other talents. For example, Kevin, who we met at the beginning of the chapter, knew his multiplication tables by age four and was drawing weather maps of all 50 states. He spoke in paragraphs at the age of 13 months, became interested in electronics between fourth and fifth grade, and was able to read diagrams and charts in books on electricity.

Hypersexuality

Hypersexuality is another symptom that can occur in some children, but it is more prevalent in adolescents with bipolar disorder. A young child, even without a history of sexual abuse or unusual exposure to sexual activities, may use language or behave in ways that are sexually provocative. Sexual profanity and excessive or even public masturbation can be observed in early childhood. Adolescents demonstrate symptoms of bipolar disorder that are closely associated with those of adults; they may be extremely sexually active and with multiple partners.[4]

Extreme Elation

Euphoria, or extreme elation, may be demonstrated by children and adolescents. Such elation may appear despite depressing or stressful circumstances. The child or adolescent may be too giddy or positive in his behavior even to recognize that his peers are not joining him in laughter. The "jokes" he presents, either verbally or by actions, may seem bizarre or beyond what others consider funny.

Hallucination

Some adolescents and young children with bipolar illness may even hallucinate. Most commonly, such hallucinations are auditory; the child or adolescent hears voices or holds imaginary conversations with another person. These conversations can be friendly, menacing, or commanding in nature. Although less typical, children can also hallucinate visually. What they think they are seeing might not be there at all, or they may be viewing extreme distortions of what is present.

Suicidal Ideation

The harsh reality is that these children and adolescents do, in fact, attempt suicide, and some succeed. Actual examples of methods tried include tying ropes or belts around their necks, cutting or poking themselves with scissors or tableware, laying behind the wheels of a parked car, or running into traffic. One of the most challenging and disturbing experiences for a parent is to witness these acts or hear their four- or five-year-old discuss jumping from a car or from the window of a tall building. Suicidal ideation is a part of the symptom profile for both adolescents and young children who suffer mood disorders. Take seriously any such discussion or any gestures toward self-injury.

Night Terrors

While it is natural for children to have the occasional nightmare, children with bipolar disorder often experience night terrors that are much more severe in their imagery. Children who are not bipolar might dream of being chased by animals or monsters, but they manage to awaken before actually being injured. Conversely, children who are bipolar dream through experiences of physical attack that involve blood and gore. These children frequently report bloody images associated with torn skin and broken bones.[5]

> *Suicidal ideation is a part of the symptom profile for both adolescents and young children who suffer mood disorders. Take seriously any such discussion or any gestures toward self-injury.*

Extreme Anxiety

Children with bipolar disorder can experience extreme anxiety. Separation anxiety in both infants and toddlers may be so severe that these children refuse to go to school. They might be extremely clingy and in need of constant reassurance. Children and adolescents may be preoccupied with death, separation, and abandonment. This anxiety may clear up with treatment, but some children require antianxiety medication.

Extreme Sensitivity to Stimuli

Children and adolescents with bipolar disorder are often extremely sensitive to stimuli. They are "thin-skinned" children who, like Brian, may be highly sensitive to touch, light, sound, taste, and/or smell.

In general, many of the symptoms of bipolar disorder in childhood and early adolescence may be reflective of an extreme lack of the capacity to self-calm, coupled with minimal-to-no tolerance of frustration. This is evidenced by the child's extremely diminished ability to regulate his affect, his quickness to become irritable and angry, his discomfort in making the slightest change in his activities, and, at times, his inability to maintain logical thought processes. During rapid-cycling or manic episodes, it may appear as if all his regulatory capacities are being challenged.

THE IMPACT OF EARLY-ONSET BIPOLAR DISORDER

The impact of bipolar illness for children and adolescents is severe and pervasive. While some children may become targets for positive attention, most are shunned or ridiculed by peers as too overbearing, aggressive, or irritable.

> The impact of bipolar illness for children and adolescents is severe and pervasive. While some children may become targets for positive attention, most are shunned or ridiculed by peers as too overbearing, aggressive, or irritable.

At home, a bipolar child draws on all of the family's emotional resources. Such children are challenging for parents as well as siblings. They need attention, special nurturing, limit-setting, and the most forgiving love. The challenge of coping with a child's bipolar illness can lead to marital conflict and divorce.

Bipolar disorder in children and adolescents competes with channeling cognitive and emotional energies essential for academic achievement. The older adolescent may have extreme difficulty continuing school.

Although a bipolar child may be extremely bright and creative in certain areas, bipolar illness interferes with a child's capacity to master skills or meet the challenges associated with normal emotional and social development.

Most alarming, bipolar illness can lead to suicide; it is a contributing factor in the significantly increasing rate of suicide among children. Between 1980 and 1992, the rate of suicide for children ages 10 to 14 increased by 120 percent.[6] In one five-year study of bipolar adolescents, 20 percent made at least one significant suicide attempt.[7]

DIAGNOSING CHILDREN AND ADOLESCENTS WITH BIPOLAR DISORDER

Diagnosing bipolar disorder in children and adolescents presents a difficult challenge. As reflected in the examples of Steve, Kevin, and Brian, a diagnosis of bipolar disorder may take years and involve numerous consultations before a correct determination is made. Specific symptoms and factors to be on the alert for include:

Frequency and rapidity of cycling from depression to mania. Young people may first present with either manic or depressive periods. Some researchers indicate that children and adolescents exhibit greater frequency and rapidity of cycling from depression to mania than do adults with bipolar disorder. Young people move from one mood to another within several days and/or several times in one day. This is described as a mixed state and can include a demonstration of each mood minutes apart or with overlap.[8]

Somber appearance, negative self-statements, suicidal threats, withdrawal, and expressions of hopelessness and helplessness. These symptoms are evidenced during depression by some children and adolescents with bipolar disorder. While children may experience euphoria, they rarely experience the extended periods of euphoria characterized by inflated self-esteem or grandiosity that are typical of adult bipolar illness. As stated earlier, their bipolar disorder is more often reflected by irritability, intense angry outbursts, physical hyperactivity, aggression, physical impulsivity, and emotional lability.

Duration of mania. Because young people often show greater emotional lability than do adults, child or adolescent mania may not often last for seven days. Rather, their moods may alternate within a day or over several days. A duration of seven days at a minimum is a defining quality for a diagnosis of bipolar disorder, according to the *Diagnostic and Statistical Manual of Mental Disorders, Fourth Edition (DSM-IV)*.[9]

Manifestation of mania. Children with mania exhibit symptoms in ways that are limited by their developmental constraints. While an adult may take trips, get involved in grandiose schemes, and run up excessive credit-card debt, children may demonstrate behavioral problems such as academic failure, fighting, dangerous risk-taking, or inappropriate sexual activity. The fact that some of these may fall within the normal range of children's behavior increases the difficulty of diagnosis.[10]

The way adolescents demonstrate evidence of mania begins to take on greater similarity to that of adults, but is still limited by the child's social and developmental boundaries. However, adolescents, more than children, may exhibit: psychotic symptoms, including mood-incongruent hallucinations, paranoia, and marked thought disorder; markedly labile moods, with mixed manic and depressive features; and severe deterioration in behavior.[11]

Children often lack the capacity to reflect on their emotional states and the language to describe their internal experiences. Self-awareness regarding one's emotional development follows a course of increasing complexity.[12] A child learns to recognize an emotion and a physical state that may correspond to it. He also learns to label his emotions with a vocabulary that takes on increasing complexity.

For example, he may initially only be able to say he feels "good" or "bad." Increased language development, an increased capacity to attend to his internal experiences, and feedback from others help him differentiate his emotions to include "sad," "mad," "happy," "jealous," and other feelings. At a more advanced level of emotional development, he may be able to identify mixed emotions, that is, feeling different ways about the same event.

Children's immaturity in language and the capacity to self-reflect clearly interferes with their being available to participate fully in a diagnostic assessment.

Traditionally, both the clinical view and the general attitude of mental health professionals prevented the assignment of the diagnosis of bipolar disorder to a child. It is human nature to minimize one's discomfort. The tendency of parents and even those in the mental health field was, and to a lesser degree still is, to regard the child's behavior as reflecting a quiet, pensive, or down mood and to ignore the severity of the symptoms. This tendency reflects an idealization of childhood that has hindered a more accurate assessment of the true clinical picture.

> *C*hildren's immaturity in language and the capacity to self-reflect clearly interferes with their being available to participate fully in a diagnostic assessment.

Likewise, professionals may dismiss mania in children and adolescents as merely indicative of the natural self-focused attention expected of children and adolescents. Mental health professionals have also been hesitant to apply the diagnosis of bipolar disorder to children and adolescents because, as stated above, the symptoms do not match those of adults diagnosed with this disorder. The descriptions of disorders in *DSM-IV* do not correspond to the symptoms evidenced by children and adolescents, but adults who are "on the edge of *DSM-IV*" may be similarly overlooked and undertreated.

Most significantly, diagnosis is often a challenge because bipolar disorder is difficult to differentiate from other diagnoses that share symptoms associated with this illness.

DIFFERENTIAL DIAGNOSIS

The major challenge in diagnosing bipolar disorder in children and adolescents is determining whether or not a child has another disorder with similar symptoms, bipolar disorder alone, or a combination of diagnoses (comorbid, or occurring together). Bipolar disorders in children and adolescents are usually a comorbid condition.

A diagnosis is based on a careful assessment of emotional, cognitive, and behavioral functioning. Taking a detailed history is important in arriving at any diagnosis, but especially when identifying bipolar illness in children and adolescents. Doctors also utilize psychological tests, urine drug screens, CAT scans of the head, and blood tests.

Attention-Deficit/Hyperactivity Disorder (ADHD)

ADHD is often difficult to distinguish from mania because of the similarity of its symptoms: impulsiveness, hyperactivity, distractibility, inattention, and irritability. Studies have indicated that many youths with bipolar disorder also have ADHD.[13] Conversely, at least 14 percent of children and adolescents with ADHD also have bipolar illness.[14] Since the cluster of symptoms associated with ADHD is often evidenced in mood disorders, a diagnosis is reached only after ruling out a mood disorder."[15]

> *While bipolar disorder affects adults of both sexes equally, studies suggest that early onset of the illness occurs more frequently in males.*

Boys are more frequently diagnosed with ADHD than are girls. Similarly, while bipolar disorder affects adults of both sexes equally, studies suggest that early onset of the illness occurs more frequently in males.[16]

In general, the symptoms appear more intense and severe when bipolar disorder is comorbid with ADHD. When these two diagnoses are not comorbid, the symptoms of ADHD are evidenced by a chronic and persistent pattern of functioning; bipolar symptoms are more erratic and severe. Bipolar symptoms, when contrasted with those of ADHD, reflect more severe difficulty in the regulation of affect (emotion), which may be reduced during periods of relative mood stability.

Important research continues to find methods to distinguish these two disorders and to identify more readily when they are comorbid. A recent study suggests the Child Behavior Checklist (CBCL) can help to make this distinction when used in conjunction with other forms of assessment. The purpose of this checklist is to assess competencies and problems of children and adolescents through ratings by observers. The checklist includes fifteen scales. Although the sample was relatively small, when parents rated their children, those with mania and ADHD had significantly higher ratings than those children with ADHD alone on the Withdrawn, Thought Problems, Delinquent Behavior, and Aggressive Behavior scales. In addition, they had higher ratings of comorbid depression, anxiety, and psychotic symptoms.[17]

Conduct Disorder

Symptoms typically the hallmark of conduct-disordered children and adolescents are also evidenced by children and adolescents who have bipolar illness. These include aggression toward people or animals, destruction of property, deceitfulness or theft, and serious violations of rules. Both disorders involve difficulties with impulse control and behavioral regulation. According to some studies, 69 percent of youths diagnosed with bipolar disorder also evidence conduct disorder at some time.[18] Conduct disorder can occur prior to the onset of bipolar disorder and subsequent to the first episode.

The key focus of study in making the differentiation of diagnosis is the presence of a repetitive and persistent pattern of the identified behaviors (in the child or adolescent with a conduct disorder) versus the more episodic or periodic demonstration of such symptoms (by the manic child or adolescent).

Unless the child or adolescent is also manic, those who have conduct disorder consistently experience less anxiety about their behaviors and appear less perplexed and less genuinely connected in their interpersonal relationships as compared to those who are manic (except during acute mania). Children and adolescents who evidence conduct disorder show long-term patterns in their lack of genuine

Bipolar disordered children and adolescents (unless also diagnosed with conduct disorder) typically express genuine remorse and guilt following incidents of aggression toward others and/or the violation of personal and social standards.

empathy for the pain of others. Bipolar disordered children and adolescents (unless also diagnosed with conduct disorder) more typically express genuine remorse and guilt following incidents of aggression toward others and/or the violation of personal and social standards. Such guilt and remorse may further compound depression in children and adolescents who have only bipolar illness.

Schizophrenia

Since adolescents with mania often have schizophrenic-like symptoms, it is difficult to distinguish an early onset of bipolar illness from the onset of schizophrenia in this age group. This is especially true when they exhibit hallucinations and delusions. Bipolar illness is more often accompanied by psychotic symptoms in children than it is in adults. The chaotic pattern of emotionality and behavior exhibited by children and adolescents with mixed states and rapid cycling also appears similar to adult schizophrenia.

Psychotic symptoms used to be considered the defining symptoms for schizophrenia; but, a distinguishing feature for those with bipolar disorder is the presence of increasing mania prior to hallucinations and delusions.

Family history is an extremely important factor to consider in distinguishing between bipolar disorder and schizophrenia.

Borderline Personality Disorder

Key features of this diagnosis may include frantic efforts to avoid real or imagined abandonment; a pattern of unstable and intense interpersonal relationships characterized by alternating between extremes of idealization and devaluation; impulsivity that is potentially self-damaging; and recurrent suicidal behaviors, gestures, threats, or self-mutilating behavior. In addition, borderline personality disorder can entail affective instability due to a marked reactivity of moods; chronic feelings of emptiness; intense anger or difficulty in controlling anger; and transient, stress-related paranoid ideation or severe dissociative symptoms.

Clearly, many of these symptoms are also part of the cluster of symptoms associated with bipolar illness. However, unless these conditions occur together, the distinguishing factor in borderline personality disorder is that these behaviors appear as part of the core personality and are pervasive and persistent. In contrast, those with bipolar illness may evidence these same behaviors, but such behaviors may stand out in sharp contrast to a more stable ongoing personality.

Substance Abuse

A major distinction between those who demonstrate behaviors due to substance abuse versus those diagnosed with bipolar illness is that the symptoms caused by substance abuse are more transient and fleeting. Such abuse may lead to euphoria, irritability, aggression, impulsivity, psychoses, or other symptoms similarly associated with child and adolescent bipolar illness. An accurate history, chemistry workup, and assessment over time are important in making this differentiation. Substance abuse is often a comorbid condition for adolescents with bipolar disorder. While substance abuse is less frequent in children, it should be emphasized that, like Danielle Steel's son Nick Traina, children may abuse over-the-counter medications.

Sexual Abuse

Children who have been sexually abused or have witnessed adult sexual behaviors often exhibit hypersexual behavior similar to that demonstrated by children with bipolar disorder. They may seem precociously preoccupied with thoughts and expressions of sexuality, demonstrate inappropriate sexual behavior, and engage in frequent self-stimulation including masturbation. A careful history and assessment over time are extremely important in making the differentiation between sexual abuse and bipolar disorder.

Differential diagnosis is a complex challenge that requires continued research to improve our ability in making an early and accurate diagnosis of bipolar disorder.

CAUSES OF EARLY-ONSET BIPOLAR DISORDER

A detailed discussion of theories regarding the etiology of adult bipolar disorder has been presented in a previous chapter. Some controversy exists concerning possible differences between the causes of early-onset versus late-onset bipolar disorder. For example, research indicates that prepubertal-onset bipolar illness is more likely associated with early aggressive hyperactivity, lithium resistance (a lack of response to lithium), and greater familial loading (frequency of presence of the disorder in the family history).[19]

Early diagnosis and prompt treatment for children suffering mood disorders are essential because individuals with early onset of the disorder are at great risk for multiple episodes of depression throughout their lifetime.

One family study of bipolar I disorder in adolescence found early-onset symptoms were linked to increased familial loading and lithium resistance.[20] Researchers are also exploring specific genetic factors that may lead to early-onset versus late-onset bipolar disorder.[21] Other studies suggest a high prevalence of alcoholism among parents of young people with mood disorders.[22]

Certain medical factors may trigger bipolar illness in children and adolescents. These include steroids taken orally, certain street drugs, and neurologic conditions such as strokes, multiple sclerosis, tumors, and epilepsy, all of which can cause symptoms that are similar to bipolar disorder.[23]

MEDICAL TREATMENT

Early diagnosis and prompt treatment for children suffering mood disorders are essential because individuals with early onset of the disorder are at great risk for multiple episodes of depression throughout their lifetime. While children and adolescents with bipolar disorder are responsive to a variety of therapies, no single definitive treatment regimen is currently available for them. Therapies used include medication, psychotherapy, family therapy, and psychoeducation.

Medication Therapy

Medication therapy is an essential component of treatment for early-onset bipolar disorder. While adults with bipolar illness may have periods of low-level depression and hypomania, children and adolescents with bipolar disorder more consistently experience severe aspects of the illness. The intensity of their mania, depression, mixed episodes, and rapid cycling demands ongoing medication management.

Each of the medications discussed below is potentially able to improve the conditions of bipolar illness. However, these drugs also have a wide range of potential side effects. The option for their usage should only be determined by knowledgeable clinicians and with the full collaboration of parents. Doctors should discuss all side effects with parents, so that they are fully informed before making essential decisions, and are also alert to possible side effects while monitoring their child's treatment. Finally, it is important not to minimize or idealize the potential of medications to produce positive change.

Lithium

Lithium has been the most consistently effective medication in the treatment of adult bipolar disorder. Approximately 80 percent of patients respond positively to lithium. It is less effective for children and adolescents, however. Although studies suggest lower success rates in

A Cautionary Note

Effective treatment depends on appropriate diagnosis of bipolar disorder in children and adolescents. There is some evidence that using antidepressant medication to treat depression in a person who has bipolar disorder may induce manic symptoms if it is taken without a mood stabilizer. In addition, using stimulant medications to treat ADHD or ADHD-like symptoms in a child with bipolar disorder may

patients taking lithium who are prone to rapid-cycling conditions of the disorder, it should be emphasized that lithium may help inhibit suicidal behavior in people with bipolar disorder.[24]

Dosage for children is similar to that for adults and, as with adults, blood levels must be carefully monitored to avoid lithium toxicity. Parents should be on the alert for possible signs of lithium toxicity, which may include: fatigue, sleepiness, confusion, hand tremor, intestinal distress, slurred speech, tremors of the lower jaw, and unsteady gait. Lithium may also cause weight gain and adolescent acne.

Nausea and vomiting are also early signs of lithium toxicity, as are mental confusion and loss of coordination. Patients who take lithium and suffer gastrointestinal illnesses resulting in vomiting or diarrhea can develop lithium toxicity from loss of sodium and potassium.

The effectiveness of lithium is usually noticed within two weeks for mania and four to six weeks for depression. While long-term use of lithium with adults has not yielded any negative effects, there are few longitudinal studies on children using lithium.

Anticonvulsant Mood Stabilizers

In recent years, a number of anticonvulsant medications have been identified as effective treatment for acute mania and the prevention of future episodes of bipolar disorder. Patients who do not respond to or who are intolerant of lithium may respond to these drugs alone or in combination with lithium. Since these anticonvulsant medications are worsen manic symptoms. While it can be hard to determine which young patients will become manic, there is a greater likelihood among children and adolescents who have a family history of bipolar disorder. If manic symptoms develop or markedly worsen during antidepressant or stimulant use, consult a physician immediately and consider a diagnosis of, and treatment for, bipolar disorder.[25]

found to be effective with rapid cycling and mixed mania, their usage with children has increased.[26] Depakote, Tegretol, Neurontin, Lamictal, Topamax, and Gabitril are most frequently prescribed for children, even though research of these drugs has concentrated more heavily on adults.[27]

Depakote can cause severe life-threatening liver toxicity, especially in children under 10 years of age. Tegretol and Lamictal can lead to life-threatening skin rashes. While these are rare side effects, it is important to bring them to the attention of the doctor as early as possible.

Antipsychotic medications are used with hesitation in children, except in extreme cases of psychosis. In adults they've been used for psychotic symptoms such as hallucinations, bizarre thinking, and unusual movements. They have also been effective for mania and mixed bipolar disorder when such psychotic symptoms are present. While each of these medications is associated with typical side effects, the newer atypical antipsychotic medications (developed since 1990) have fewer side effects. One of these atypical antipsychotic medications, Zyprexa, has been recently approved by the FDA for active mania.

Sedatives

This group of medications has been found to quiet people while diminishing anxiety and activity and fostering a more normal sleep pattern. This is especially significant in light of studies indicating that

Electroconvulsive Therapy (ECT) for Children

ECT, which has undergone significant change and refinement over the years, has been found to be as effective a treatment for children and adolescents as it is for adults. Excellent results have been observed in some young people who have severe depression, psychosis, suicidal ideation, and mania that are minimally or unresponsive to medication.

ECT in children is rarely used, however, and only in extreme cases, as when the child has failed to respond to all other known treatments.

the normalizing of sleep patterns can greatly reduce frequency of mania (see chapter 4).

Antidepressants

While antidepressants are invaluable in the treatment of unipolar depression, increasing research suggests they may actually be detrimental when treating children and adults for bipolar disorder during depressive episodes. Specifically, the administration of antidepressants during depressive episodes can trigger an attack of mania. This risk is much greater if the patient is not receiving a mood-stabilizing agent.

In one study of 120 children with bipolar disorder, more than 80 percent escalated into full-blown mania, psychosis, or aggressive behavior following the administration of antidepressant medications.[28] For this reason, these need to be used cautiously and with close monitoring.

Psychotherapy

Psychotherapy is an essential complement in the effective treatment of child and adolescent bipolar disorder. Such therapy takes a number of forms, including individual therapy, group therapy, couples therapy, family therapy, and multiple-family therapy. Parents and patient may engage in any one of these treatments or in several treatments simultaneously.

Individual Therapy

Individual psychotherapy may be indicated for the child or adolescent with bipolar illness. A necessary prerequisite for such participation is that he is sufficiently stabilized to make use of such treatment. In the context of individual therapy, a child or adolescent may be helped to explore his emotions and attitudes about his illness. He can be helped to develop an increased capacity to reflect on the details of his experience so

> In one study of 120 children with bipolar disorder, more than 80 percent escalated into full-blown mania, psychosis, or aggressive behavior following the administration of antidepressant medications.

that he can become engaged, whenever possible, as an observer of the course of his illness. He may similarly learn strategies for monitoring his behavior so as to maximize his capacity, in light of his illness, for recognizing depressive thoughts, irritability, anger, and other subjective experiences that accompany bipolar disorder. Individual therapy can also facilitate his compliance with medications, a major challenge in the treatment of bipolar disorder in both children and adults.

Individual therapy may be indicated for each parent as well, to help each of them deal with the personal impact of the illness. This may especially be indicated when a couple is simultaneously involved in couples therapy and when one partner is more severely affected by the child's illness.

Group Therapy

Children and adolescents with bipolar illness may be encouraged to become involved in group therapy or a support group in which they have the opportunity to feel connected to others coping with the same challenge. As with individual treatment, such participation is only feasible when sufficient stabilization has been achieved.

Couples Therapy

In this form of psychotherapy, couples are encouraged to share candidly their reactions to the intense demands of having a child with bipolar disorder. The relationship of couples who have a child with special needs is a relationship that is extremely challenged. This is especially true when the special need involves bipolar disorder.

> The chronic display of extremely difficult behavior demands constant attention and has a direct impact on all of the family resources and, indeed, on the stability of the marriage.

The chronic display of extremely difficult behavior demands constant attention and has a direct impact on all of the family resources and, indeed, on the stability of the marriage. Facing this challenge often causes parents to feel helpless and ashamed and, subsequently, to isolate from others and each other. This is a time that calls for improved communication, sharing, and mutual support and nurturance. It is a time when such illness can lead to individual isolation resulting from guilt, anger, shame, a sense of inadequacy, and, perhaps most important, a sense of helplessness. If the parents are to be effectively available to help their child, they need to be helped to be available to each other.

Family Therapy

There may be times when the entire family, including the child with bipolar illness, will meet in special session. These periodic meetings help to foster candid communication, allow family members to share how they are impacted, identify family strengths, and develop new ways of responding to this exceptional challenge. Family therapy is especially beneficial when siblings are involved. Participation by the child with bipolar disorder is indicated if he or she is emotionally available and can be an active participant in the process. Since this demands a level of stability and a capacity to deal with such sharing, such participation should be carefully evaluated.

Family-Focused Psychoeducation

As described in the previous chapter, family-focused psychoeducation may be indicated to help the family develop new skills in communication, problem solving, and stress management. This is especially important when dealing with children and adolescents with bipolar disorder. Siblings and other caretakers can also be involved in such treatment in order to develop consistency in the approaches used.

Family-focused education is a powerful tool in improving negative expressed emotion (EE). Research with bipolar disorder has identified negative EE—a critical attitude toward patients on the part of family members—as a crucial variable that can lead to a poor treatment outcome. Addressing negative expressed emotion in family therapy and in family-focused education may have a significant impact on medication compliance, and foster appropriate sleep patterns and overall adherence to the treatment program.

All family members, including the child with bipolar disorder (when stable and of an appropriate age), benefit by learning cognitive-behavioral and behavioral methods that can be used with children to help them increase self-control regarding attention, impulsiveness, and anger management. Families can similarly be assisted in learning strategies to help them respond to the intense aggression that such children demonstrate.

Knowledge about recognizing and managing symptoms, treatment approaches, criteria for hospitalization, and how to facilitate hospitalization, when necessary, are just a few of the issues that can be addressed in this context.

Multiple-Family Therapy

This form of therapy was first practiced with families of psychiatrically hospitalized patients. Therapists meet with many families of patients in a large group. This format allows for increased support by sharing general information and strategies to help families cope with bipolar disorder.

Support Groups

While support groups are extremely helpful for adults with bipolar disorder, support groups for parents of children with bipolar disorder should be considered a necessary component of the treatment plan. Meeting and sharing with other parents who are similarly challenged by the trauma of this illness helps to provide knowledge and support while reducing the intense sense of isolation that so often accompanies caring for a child or adolescent with bipolar disorder. Some groups focus on support or advocacy and others serve both functions. You can find a support group by contacting your local mental health center, hospital social services, health-care professional organizations, Child and Adolescent Bipolar Foundation (CABF), and National DMDA, or through Internet Web sites. CABF offers free online parent support groups (see appendix: "Resources for Information").

> While support groups are extremely helpful for adults with bipolar disorder, support groups for parents of children with bipolar disorder should be considered a necessary component of the treatment plan.

NEW HOPE

In spite of this most complex and challenging disorder, new hope exists for parents and their children. Recent developments offer increased hope for earlier recognition, accurate diagnosis, and effective treatment and management of early-onset bipolar disorder. The following are some of these hopeful developments:

1. Increased awareness of early-onset bipolar disorder has led to new research regarding those medications most effective in the treatment of children and adolescents.

2. Medical and mental health professionals are being educated in greater numbers regarding diagnosis and treatment of an illness that, until recently, was rarely considered for children and adolescents.

3. New forms of psychoeducation are being identified in an effort to promote stabilization.

4. Mental health and professional organizations are increasingly advocating for parity of mental health with physical health in insurance coverage.

5. The Internet allows rapid access of information and facilitates communication among all people involved in living with bipolar illness. This has enabled families (parents, children, and adolescents) to feel less isolated. A connection of support to meet the challenges of living with bipolar disorder is readily available.

6. Associations such as the Child and Adolescent Bipolar Foundation have formed to provide parents with a range of services, including education, support, and advocacy.

SUMMARY

The family with a child who has a bipolar illness is continually challenged, 24 hours a day, seven days a week. And yet the family is only one small part of a much larger community that needs to unite with help and support in a collaborative effort to meet this challenge. The combined effort of family and community in reaching out to help children with bipolar disorder is the philosophy behind C.A.R.E. (compassion, advocacy, recognition, and education).

CHAPTER 11

Living with People with Bipolar Disorder

WHAT IMAGE DO we portray to other people? If we could peer into a mirror and see our true reflection, could we accept what we see as truthful? Many of us might be surprised, and even shocked, to discover that our self-image is quite different from the image we project to others.

A quick glance in the mirror each morning gives us a surface impression, like the jacket cover of a book, but we cannot envision how others perceive us any more clearly than we can hear the tone of our own voice when we speak. Have you ever been startled by the way you sound on a tape recording of your voice? Moreover, everyone's perception is different because no two people view the same object or situation equally. The question remains, What is reality?

Each of us constructs a self-image, a defining personality that includes internal guidelines or standards by which we assess how to think, feel, and behave. Some of us develop guidelines that permit a lot of space and freedom, that give us room to feel, think, and behave. If we are flexible in our guidelines, this permits a greater range for self-expression. A lack of guidelines or too much flexibility leaves us subject to whim and inherent confusion, both for ourselves and others.

More rigid guidelines, on the other hand, lead to great trepidation when coming close to the self-applied limits, and even greater anxiety, guilt, or shame if such guideposts are crossed.

Personal standards are based on a variety of factors that influence personality. These factors include genetic predisposition, messages one might have heard growing up, and modeling after mentors. In addition, occupation, religion, gender, age, ethnicity, culture, and socioeconomic level all influence and provide a basis for the standards by which we live. For example, a teacher might expect to conform to certain guidelines that are acceptable within the parameters of her profession. People often follow standards of behavior based on their religion.

> Our reactions to other people give us more insight into ourselves than into others. If we choose only to focus on the behavior of others, we will get to know how they behave. If we focus on how we are influenced by others and look still further inward, we will more clearly recognize our inner self.

Public reaction to George Bush's parachute jump several years ago reflects a range of personal standards. Some reacted with strong annoyance, declaring that he should "act his age." Others applauded his efforts to redefine the parameters of how a senior could be spending time. Some watch movies of Robin Williams or Roberto Benigni and consider both actors "off the wall," while others are envious of their passion and energy.

Our reactions to other people give us more insight into ourselves than into others. If we choose only to focus on the behavior of others, we will get to know how they behave. If we focus on how we are influenced by others and look still further inward, we will more clearly recognize our inner self.

Witnessing the behavior of someone with bipolar disorder, particularly during severe manic or depressive episodes, forces us to visit the boundaries of our own personalities. While this may occur in the context of any relationship, such an experience is intensified in a close relationship with someone who is bipolar.

If people have conflicting feelings or are sensitive about their own spontaneity, they may experience heightened tension in a relationship with someone who is manic. For example, if your anxiety level escalates when you pursue a dream or feel uninhibited, you may experience tension in such a relationship and begin to question your guidelines. Other people, due to their own uneasiness about attention-seeking behavior, may feel discomfort when observing aspects of manic behavior that elicit attention for someone with bipolar illness.

RECOGNIZING THE INNER SELF

Manic behavioral moods—grandiose and uninhibited thinking—may lead patients to the very brink of their own impulses until they are forced

> Witnessing the behavior of someone with bipolar disorder forces us to visit the boundaries of our own personalities. While this may occur in the context of any relationship, such an experience is intensified in a close relationship with someone who is bipolar.

to confront and define themselves. Observers might feel comfortable, if certain manic behaviors resonate with their own, until a patient goes "too far." Most people can be objective in assessing when "too far" is clearly destructive. Even mild mania may be threatening, however, if observers perceive such behavior as beyond their own limits, dangerous, "bad," "not me," or if observers are fearful and somewhat anxious about their own dreams and hopes. Those unafflicted will similarly experience tension if mania stirs up their yearnings about being more uninhibited and spontaneous, especially if they are questioning their self-imposed limitations.

If you are an acquaintance of someone who is bipolar, it is easier to set limits and keep the relationship narrowly defined. If you are trying to maintain a deeper intimacy, however, you must expect some underlying tension. You may need to define specific guidelines for yourself regarding your relationship and how you will respond to the tension. If you don't set these guidelines, you may tend to react rather than act.

As in any relationship, the more prone we are to react without a real sense of choice, the more we feel overly influenced by the other person. This is another reason why you might wish to define your own thinking if you're involved in an intimate relationship with someone who is bipolar. Communicating these guidelines out loud is secondary to establishing clear guidelines for yourself because the person with bipolar illness may, or may not, be able to respect such limits, depending on the severity of symptoms.

If a friend or loved one suffers from severe depression, be forewarned that the impact of being around someone who is emotionally constricted can cause you grief. You may experience a mild sense of hopelessness and helplessness. Increased tension is possible, especially if a part of you shares any propensity to depressive moods. It is also possible that your relationship with a severely depressed loved one may bring on your worst anxieties, self-doubts, and pessimism.

> As in any relationship, the more prone we are to react without a real sense of choice, the more we feel overly influenced by the other person.

Although tension may be a natural reaction, you may be less affected by someone's depression or mania if you are comfortable and secure with yourself. You still feel empathy, but you don't feel threatened by the other person's state. You might still want to set limits, both in terms of time spent together and the level of intimacy desired.

Always be prepared for a more intense and intimate relationship with someone who is bipolar. In the context of such intimacy, you will be confronted with a very different set of expectations. You may even feel pushed to the edge of your "defined" personality.

KNOW THYSELF

As mentioned earlier, our feelings toward others—our likes, dislikes, attractions, irritations, admiration, and our repulsion—tell us more about ourselves than about others. Our reactions inform us of our passions, hopes, needs, expectations, longings, anxieties, and fears. They are mere reflections of our inner selves.

While the maxim "know thyself" has in recent decades increasingly become a part of American culture, it is especially important if you are in a relationship with someone who has bipolar illness. Whether you are a spouse, parent, son or daughter, sibling, colleague, or friend, your relationship is bound to be a challenging one. It may lead to feelings of excitement and frustration, joy and anger, fear and resentment, a sense of contentment or a sense of dread. Within the relationship, you may feel strongly connected one moment and estranged

> *Always be prepared for a more intense and intimate relationship with someone who is bipolar. In the context of such intimacy, you will be confronted with a very different set of expectations. You may even feel pushed to the very edge of your "defined" personality.*

at another. Overall, you may feel trusted and accepted, but at times feel devalued and rejected. You may even experience that well-known stress response of "fight or flight": on one hand, wanting to leave, but on the other, wanting to strike back. In the midst of all this, you are trying to sort out your guilt, your own needs, and the needs of your loved one.

Despite the fact that most relationships encompass many of these reactions and issues, you may feel more vulnerable in a relationship with someone who has bipolar illness because of the unpredictable and intense nature of the disorder. While a sense of vulnerability may not necessarily arise during those weeks, months, or even years when the disorder is stabilized, it is likely to be triggered when your loved one is experiencing intense depression or mania. Knowing yourself is your best defense.

Becoming in tune with your feelings results from working toward a greater understanding of your own sensitivities to depression and mania. We all possess these predispositions. The uniqueness of your individual personality influences how you respond to these extremes of behavior. For some, depression may be a familiar feeling because of a propensity to experience depressed moods. Biology and family history, which may include manic or depressive episodes, trauma, or other similar experiences, contribute to these sensitivities. Even if you've grown up in a nurturing and positive environment (and are not reacting based on your own insecurities or unresolved issues), you may tend to adopt the more universally held beliefs, e.g., "the stigma," regarding behavior associated with manic-depressive illness. These attitudes and sensitivities frequently surface when living with someone with bipolar illness.

> While the maxim "know thyself" has in recent decades increasingly become a part of American culture, it is an especially important aspiration if you are in a relationship with someone who has bipolar illness.

By knowing yourself, you can see more clearly how your needs, fears, and expectations are impacted when confronted with depression or mania. Likewise, knowledge offers you a greater capacity to respond to and manage your reactions. You can more objectively assess your contribution to the relationship, react less intensely, and learn to recognize choices and make clear decisions. It is important to identify those aspects of the relationship over which you can exert some control and those over which you have little or no control. If you prioritize your needs, it is fair to expect your partner to honor those that are most important to you.

Similarly, you need to examine your expectations of the relationship and determine which ones are realistic and which are unrealistic. With this knowledge, you can maintain a greater sense of stability while living with a person with bipolar illness. Without this knowledge, your relationship is more likely to arouse self-doubt and related internal and interpersonal friction.

In general, people tend to respond favorably to someone with low-level mania. The very traits that are symptomatic of hypomania—energy, drive, optimism, and lack of inhibitions—are also components of healthy, optimal living. In the presence of a person with hypomania, it is possible to feel more confident and energized, and to learn to take action as we strive toward the fulfillment of our own dreams. The qualities exhibited during low-level mania are contagious and resonate with the part of ourselves that fosters trust. Leadership ability and creativity are exemplified characteristics of low-level mania (hypomania). It is this very energy that has inspired many artists and world leaders.

How we react in a relationship with someone who has bipolar illness greatly depends on the context of that relationship as well as our own needs and expectations. Take, for example, a patient by the name of Mark who reported a gradual shift in his feelings toward his wife over a three-year period.

When Mark first met Rachel, she was a real-estate agent, and he was immediately attracted to her gregariousness, high energy level, effervescent demeanor, and physical attractiveness. He reported that he felt "so alive" in her presence because she was "spontaneous, free spirited, and zany." Ironically, one year after their marriage, Mark's major complaint about Rachel was that she became "too outgoing, too gregarious, too free spirited, and too spontaneous." In the context of marriage, and partially as the result of his own anxieties and insecurities, Mark's needs and expectations of Rachel shifted. Again, it is easy to place all of the blame on bipolar disorder. In actuality, it is not uncommon for the very qualities that first attracted us to someone to end up repelling us.

> You need to examine your expectations of the relationship and determine which ones are realistic and which are unrealistic. Without this knowledge, your relationship is more likely to arouse self-doubt and related internal and interpersonal friction.

Like Mark, people who are intense about feeling "in control" may experience related fears that result in their inability to be self-trusting in a close relationship with someone who displays even low-level mania. The consequence of such a relationship might lead to severe tension and anxiety. In this context, strongly motivated people may

Denial and Enabling

Sometimes the healthy partner's approach is to neglect to notice any signs of the stricken partner's illness. Consciously or unconsciously, it is possible to minimize, ignore, or even fail to see symptoms when in denial. We may even conspire with someone who has bipolar disorder by failing to acknowledge the illness and promoting the avoidance of seeking and maintaining treatment.

feel threatened and take action to safeguard their own sense of security by stifling the first sign of manic behavior in the other person.

Author John Gray (*Men Are from Mars, Women Are from Venus*) suggests that men and women come from different places in approaching their needs and expectations of their relationships. Gray's viewpoint emphasizes that women tend to focus a lot of emotional energy on and feel responsible for maintaining harmony in their relationships. Given this, if the woman with bipolar disorder assumes a more active role and has a tendency to overvalue her contribution to the relationship by insisting on harmony at all cost, the relationship becomes more challenging and stressful for the healthy partner when problems arise. To know oneself, therefore, involves recognition of one's strengths, weaknesses, and limitations. We need to be realistic in our self-appraisal and in our ability to contribute to and influence the tone of a relationship.

SELF-ABSORPTION

A major aspect of bipolar illness, self-absorption strongly influences relationships. In severe depression, the afflicted are constricted in thoughts, emotions, and behavior. They have little energy and must conserve whatever emotional resources that do exist. As we have stated throughout this book, depression brings forth feelings of hope-

In studying alcoholism, researchers have termed this process "enabling." This term is equally relevant to our understanding of bipolar relationships. The ultimate impact of such apparent neglect is that the individual with bipolar illness and the relationship suffer equal damage.

lessness and helplessness. Increased self-disparagement and a sense of futility, shame, and dread foster further self-preoccupation. When the intensity level and frequency of these thoughts and emotions take precedent in the focus of their attention, depressed people are less available to listen to others, show empathy, or even be involved with loved ones.

As we have seen in other chapters, people with extreme forms of mania are predisposed to self-absorption, but are not marked by hopelessness and helplessness. On the contrary, extreme mania is punctuated by tremendous activity as well as thoughts that go in many different directions. In the extreme, self-absorption may involve distracting psychotic thoughts in which inner voices or delusions take the forefront of attention. People in this state experience real relationships as mere distractions unless they can help further their needs and dreams.

> People who are intense about feeling "in control" may experience related fears that result in their inability to be self-trusting in a close relationship with someone who displays even low-level mania.

Even low-level manic-depressives tend to be self-absorbed. This becomes a challenge for friends and loved ones who want to understand and manage their own feelings, but are blocked in their attempt because of the afflicted ones' reduced availability for interpersonal relationships.

If you are a friend or loved one of someone who suffers from bipolar illness, you may experience a deep sense of loss as the severity of symptoms increases. The dynamics of the relationship shift as the afflicted person becomes less available than before the symptoms surfaced. Increasing self-absorption may produce such a shift in personality that you feel as though the person you loved is no longer there. This shift and your sense of loss may not be as intense when the depression or mania is at a mild level. As symptoms worsen, so does your sense of loss.

> If you are a friend or loved one of someone who suffers from bipolar illness, you may experience a deep sense of loss as the severity of symptoms increases.

While this loss is not comparable to losing someone to death, there are some similarities in the feelings involved.

If we first understand ourselves, we are then in a better place to manage our loss. The second step involves learning how to deal with this change.

A major goal in working with people with manic-depression is to help them accept the reality of their illness. Those of us who have relationships with people with the disorder need to learn how to manage our own part of the relationship constructively and to acknowledge and accept feelings we experience in reaction to bipolar illness.

Whether we feel loss, resentment, frustration, or anxiety, it is only by identifying our reactions that we can experience a greater understanding and control over how we respond to this changing relationship. For example, in our reaction to the loss associated with self-absorption, we might only recognize anger and not see the grief. Or we might personalize the situation and feel depressed over what we perceive to be our contribution to such self-absorption or neglect. It is also possible to go on "automatic pilot" and adopt the role of a parent rather than a caretaker. You may ruminate over what you perceive to be a personal weakness in your loved one and the fact that somehow your advice is no longer needed. Or you may worry about your loved one looking elsewhere for excitement and stimulation.

If you are prone to self-talk and tune in, you might hear, "If only I say the right thing, then maybe he'll go for a medication assessment; if he cared for me more, he would be motivated to spend more time with me instead of on his many projects; I was too involved with my career and didn't pay enough attention to him." While any one of these comments may reflect some reality during the more stable phase of the relationship, they are far less relevant in accounting for the reality of a relationship with someone in the throes of intense mania or depression.

In recent years, researchers have been exploring the role of attention deficit disorder (ADD) in adults and how this disorder affects relationships. These studies provide an alternative view of self-absorption. As an illustration, here is the story of a couple who Bernie counseled several years ago.

Linda presented complaints that her husband, Peter, was constantly self-absorbed. She described him being late for appointments, not listening to her, and even forgetting her birthday for two consecutive years. In spite of numerous complaints, his continued self-absorption led her to feel that he no longer cared for her. One view of Peter's lack of capacity to attend to Linda is that he was self-absorbed by his own needs, selfish, unable to be empathic with another human being, self-centered, and self-focused. Some might describe him as "narcissistic." However, research now suggests that adults, like children, experience ADD. This information allowed Linda to consider a different meaning for Peter's behavior, which she could then use in evaluating whether it was a genuine lack of caring or his heightened distractibility that made him unavailable to her.

> It is helpful to recognize that the self-absorption of your partner, colleague, or friend may not be a reaction to you but a reaction to bipolar illness.

In a parallel way, it is helpful to recognize that the self-absorption of your partner, colleague, or friend may not be a reaction to you but a reaction to bipolar illness. While we have emphasized that bipolar illness distracts one from being available, it should be emphasized that any individual has a unique personality aside from being bipolar. The ability to be available, to be empathic and caring, is best reflected during a person's more stable moods. Moreover, we should acknowledge the presence of many other factors that contribute to one's capacity for intimacy.

Perhaps the most difficult part for the healthy person involved is in trying to gauge which part of a person's character may be due to bipolar illness as distinguished from their "normal" or baseline personality. If someone is narcissistic by nature, then being bipolar may only accentuate this characteristic.

COPING STRATEGIES

In addition to knowing yourself and understanding the dynamics of a relationship with someone who has bipolar illness, other factors that can further improve your sense of well-being as you cope with this challenging task include stress management, creating your own support system, psychotherapy or counseling, psychoeducation, educating yourself about bipolar disorder, and developing a list of resources for information and services.

Stress Management

Whether you are a friend or a family member of someone with bipolar illness, you are experiencing stress. It may be in the form of tension in communication, a loss in the quality of the relationship, or difficulties in being assertive. You may also experience stress related to role changes, the pressures of caretaking, financial pressure, stigma, lost income, and the emotional stress of coping with someone in a depressed or manic state.

Stress management is essential for nurturing you while someone you love is ill. It should involve some of the guidelines that we generally associate with stress management, but also focus on the specific stress of living with someone with bipolar. Techniques include learning new skills regarding time management, learning to care for the caretaker, physical relaxation strategies, maintaining your own life (friends, hobbies, your own activities), developing and practicing assertiveness skills, and maintaining healthy nutritional and physical well-being.

Maintaining balance in your life is difficult enough even during the best of times. Responding to a loved one who has bipolar illness can be all-consuming, especially during severe manic or depressive episodes. Whether you are concerned about the suicidal potential in periods of intense depression, or psychotic reactions to financial ruin or legal involvement as fallout of severe mania, living with a loved one with bipolar illness draws on all of your energies and resources and can put the relationship to the test.

> *Maintaining balance in your life is difficult enough even during the best of times. Responding to a loved one who has bipolar illness can be all-consuming, especially during severe manic or depressive episodes.*

Being able to continue attending to your needs is a priority for your own emotional balance as well as for being available to support your loved one. It is easily stated, and universally challenging during the more stressful periods, but perhaps the best strategy to practice in coping with this situation is to make sure you have a personal support system.

Create and Maintain a Personal Support System

As much as your inclination might be to isolate yourself, the best strategy you can employ in living with someone with bipolar illness is to create and maintain a personal support system. Maintaining ties with friends and relatives serves a variety of purposes. When you are experiencing a sense of isolation and loss, keeping connections is especially important. Maintaining contacts with people who you genuinely trust offers you emotional support and an objective view when your own objectivity may be decreasing because of the emotional strain. Support is also essential for your self-esteem, which can decrease in reaction to this challenge.

Having people available to do errands and help out with some of the chores of daily living, especially during periods of exacerbation of symptoms, is another reason for maintaining connections and having a support system in place.

Psychotherapy and Counseling

Psychotherapy and counseling can provide you not only greater understanding of how to live more constructively with a loved one who has bipolar illness, but also how to better recognize, make sense of, and manage the wide range of reactions you will experience in this context. Whether you seek couples counseling, family therapy, or individual treatment, such involvement offers constructive ways of living with bipolar illness.

Just as we suggest that you interview several psychiatrists regarding medication treatment for someone with bipolar illness, we strongly recommend that you interview several therapists for your own psychotherapy or counseling. Your major priorities in making your choice should be the quality of the rapport as well as the experience a particular therapist has in addressing the issues you are facing.

Psychoeducation

Family-focused psychoeducation is another approach that shows much promise in helping relatives (parents or spouse) live with bipolar illness. While these programs were originally found to be highly successful family treatments for schizophrenia, they have now been adapted to help families cope with bipolar illness. The following assumptions can be made for both illnesses:[1]

1. An episode of a psychiatric disorder represents a severe environmental challenge to a family system;

2. In response to such episodes, families often become disorganized in ways that may inhibit the patient's recovery. Communication and

problem-solving skills that were previously practiced are ignored during the period of acute illness, especially within families in which tensions were previously present.

3. Family-focused psychoeducation can assist in achieving a new state of equilibrium.

Psychoeducation programs include educating the family unit about bipolar disorder, its signs and symptoms, and its etiology and treatment. Most significantly, families are helped to learn communication skills (training in active listening, delivering positive and negative verbal feedback, and requesting changes in the behavior of the other family members) and problem-solving skills (identifying problems, generating and evaluating solutions, and implementing solutions) that help foster stabilization and may inhibit relapses.

In part, these programs are based on research findings indicating that intense levels of emotional expression are associated with stressful patterns of interaction between bipolar patients and their relatives during the post-episode period. Expressed emotion in these studies refers to critical, hostile, or overinvolved attitudes that relatives maintain toward a family member with a psychiatric disorder. Families who received family-focused psychoeducational therapy have been found to exhibit more positive interactional

> Families who received family-focused psychoeducational therapy have been found to exhibit more positive interactional behavior, and patients have evidenced reductions in mood disorder symptoms when assessed one year after treatment.

behavior (specifically nonverbal behavior), and patients have evidenced reductions in mood disorder symptoms, when assessed one year after treatment. Research in this area continues to try to identify those skills that may be most effective with specific types of families.[2]

Education

An extremely significant strategy for living with a loved one who has bipolar illness is to educate yourself about the illness. As emphasized throughout this book, knowledge offers strength. Learning how to recognize symptoms, keeping current of new medications, and developing awareness about support services and advocacy groups are all ways to educate yourself about mood disorders.

In addition to books that offer a clinical focus, reading biographies of people with bipolar disorder can lead you to a greater understanding of the illness through the personal disclosures and perspectives of those afflicted with it. Increasingly, those who live with someone with bipolar illness are sharing their experiences. Reading these accounts can help restore your sense of connection and ease the isolation you may feel in responding to this illness.

Developing a List of Resources

In helping you to cope with a friend or loved one with bipolar illness, it is important to gather a wide variety of resources. These may include educational groups, names of support agencies, books, and videotapes. Such resources have increased in recent years and offer invaluable aid, in terms of information on available services and on dealing with every aspect of mood disorders.

Do your research in your community to help you identify medical doctors who treat bipolar illness. Afterwards, interview several doctors to determine with whom you feel the most rapport. In addition, inquire as to what percentage of their practice involves actual treatment of individuals with bipolar illness.

Since we have witnessed great advances in the treatment of mood disorders, your best choices of doctors are those who frequently treat this illness. These specialists will have the most up-to-date information about prescribing medications that might work best for specific symptoms and for each individual.

Bear in mind that close supervision of any medical therapy is extremely important, particularly during the initial period of treatment. Frequent monitoring should involve face-to-face contact between the patient and the doctor to determine the effect of a specific drug and its dosage on the individual.

We strongly recommend careful research even if your loved one refuses treatment. If you wait for a crisis to occur before seeking help, it may be too late.

Your list of resources should include crisis assistance in the event your loved one needs medical attention and psychological help. While you may never require this assistance, you will feel prepared if you have these phone numbers on hand.

As part of your research, you may also want to inquire into the services psychiatric facilities in your community provide for people with mood disorders. Learn which procedures are necessary to follow should you become so concerned that you need to commit your loved one to a psychiatric setting. Such agencies may provide support services in the form of education, self-help groups, and family therapy for both the healthy partners and family members as well as those afflicted with bipolar illness.

NANCY PROBES FOR ANSWERS

In order to understand how I, as a manic-depressive, affect others living around me I asked for candid responses. "Be honest," I urged. "This is a book about truth. I'm taking a hard look at myself; no pretenses permitted." The result has been an "out-of-body" experience for me, as I needed to step back and clinically reflect on the findings of my research without permitting emotion to dominate my thoughts.

Lois: Empathy and Unconditional Friendship

My friend Lois was somewhat hesitant because, as she honestly admitted, she felt uncertain about exploring such feelings.

"We've been friends for a long time, Nancy, but some things I feel uneasy about delving into. Over the years I have sometimes reacted positively, and at other times negatively, to various situations you've related to me. I carry these thoughts around with me while considering all aspects, both positive and negative. But regardless of how I personally feel about any one particular incident, what matters most is that our friendship is unconditional."

Although Lois internalizes a lot of what I confide in her, she also is forthright with her feelings and responses. If I happen to be at the height of a manic episode, she may defer saying something to me so as not to add fuel to the fire. When she feels that I'm in a good place to listen, she'll say, "I hear you, but I don't understand. I think you're making a mistake. I wish you'd reconsider."

"What I admire most is your willingness to accept criticism, and your desire to change," said Lois. "You look for honesty in relationships, and I respect this. What's so reassuring is that we can level with each other without worrying about offending one another. This is what makes our friendship special."

> Lois is sensitive to my bipolar condition. She has never minimized it or ridiculed me for my actions, which at times I know can be difficult to deal with.

I have known Lois for more than 30 years, since we were classmates in high school. As we matured, so has our friendship. We recognize and accept each other's strengths and limitations, and from this has emerged a deep mutual respect and sisterly loyalty. Lois is sensitive to my bipolar condition. She has never minimized it or ridiculed me for my actions, which at times I know can be difficult to deal with. When I become too intense, she tells me about it.

Dianna: Setting Limits and Applying the Brakes

Frequently, Dianna Bolen, my coauthor for *Just as Much a Woman*, would caution me, "Slow down. Focus, Nancy. Focus!" Dianna described me as "charming and glowing with energy," but she has often backed away because these very symptoms make her feel off-balance and uneasy.

While collaborating on our book, Dianna and I used to enjoy periodic get-togethers over a few glasses of wine as we talked business. We became personal friends and confidants.

"When you describe an event, it's reflected both in your tone and rate of speech, as if something big is about to happen," said Dianna. "There's an aura of excitement around you, but as we sit for long periods I feel disjointed, somehow distant, like I'm viewing a special effects scene at a movie theater. I'm drawn into the drama, yet not fully a part." Dianna became edgy when I "rambled." She also commented about feeling "a twinge of sadness" although she did not understand why. "Is it me?" she asked herself, "or is it something about Nancy?"

During the drive home after one of our luncheon meetings, Dianna told me that her mind began to wander as she reflected on her afternoon experience. "I began with what I knew to be true," she mused, "that I am an outgoing, enthusiastic person with plenty of energy. But with you I felt kind of 'slow.'"

In time, Dianna began to grow weary of my apparent highs and lows and, likewise, I became increasingly disenchanted by what I considered to be her insensitivity to my affliction. This dilemma became more and more upsetting for me, and my agitation escalated still further while my self-confidence temporarily eroded.

When we reached the final editing stages of *Just as Much a Woman,* our work pace quickened. As primary author and literary agent, I phoned Dianna more regularly during this period. Dianna's translation of my communications was "trivial details unrelated to the book." She felt that my messages carried a "sense of urgency" and that my points were sometimes "repetitive." I am accustomed to replying immediately to telephone messages, faxes, and e-mail correspondence. Dianna, on the other hand, gives herself a 24-hour window for response. That works for her, but annoys me. It seemed clear that Dianna and I had different ideas about what is "important." My manner of dealing was to wait an hour or two and if she didn't call/fax back, I sometimes repeated the message if I felt it was important and could not wait. Is it possible, I thought, that heightened tension has prompted Dianna to hold the relationship with me at bay by keeping it narrowly defined? Apparently, she had begun to distance herself.

Finally, Dianna attempted to structure our conversations so they did not exceed 10 to 15 minutes. I found this restriction exasperating. What had gotten into her, I thought? Where is her flexibility? Isn't "flexibility" the name of the game? Since when does she have the right to place restrictions on me? How insulting!

"What's your goal, Nancy?" Dianna would ask. Frequent clashes resulted because it is difficult and unnatural for me to talk "bottom line." I envisioned an imaginary time clock, and in order to get in all my thoughts I began to talk faster and faster.

Several months after Dianna and I had completed working on the book, she described her thoughts in a short personal essay: "Nancy is speaking louder and faster. Her voice is strident, the sweetness gone. How does she have time to breathe between words? She accuses me of being critical of her. I feel I am not being heard. In frustration, I put down the phone and walk away. When I return a few minutes later, Nancy is still talking; she did not even notice my absence.

> *Finally, Dianna attempted to structure our conversations so they did not exceed 10 to 15 minutes. I envisioned an imaginary time clock, and in order to get in all my thoughts I began to talk faster and faster.*

"It's Tuesday afternoon and my answering machine is blinking to be played. My fax machine is spewing out pages sent by Nancy. I let out a sigh and ignore the faxes. I have received hundreds of faxes from Nancy at all hours of the day and night. Many times, there is no new information. Or I receive six faxes of the same form letter, each addressed to a different recipient. I despise the wastefulness. I resent the intrusiveness. I am angry."

Stepping aside, I can now see how Dianna's frustration over this matter must have heated up to the point of actual boiling. But I, too, was at the brink of explosion. We are two strong-willed individuals who have different priorities and working styles that were just not meshing.

Over a period of months, our relationship eroded still further. While we continued professionally, we otherwise kept at a comfortable distance. I wondered if this was another ending. Here I was again, experiencing heightened tension with a friend who was distancing, setting limits, and applying brakes.

Yuri: Visiting the Boundaries and Returning to Friendship

I had gone through that kind of distancing with Yuri, but we survived many endings and many new beginnings.

My relationship with Yuri has manifested extremes at every level because of the intimate quality of our friendship. Since he has observed me at close range during episodes of mania and severe depression, Yuri has been forced to visit the boundaries of his own personality. When Yuri feels threatened by the intensity of my mood swings, he slams on the brakes and takes off in flight. "I'm off to Australia," he'll announce. "Don't find me!" This sudden distancing leaves me bereft, exacerbating my already high level of anxiety, and I engage in irrational, sometimes dangerous, behavior.

Yuri and I had formed an intimate relationship "of sorts" as we struggled from 1982 to 1987 from both sides of the Iron Curtain for his freedom and right to exist. In response to my information gathering for this book on how my illness affected those around me, he said, "You know my answer. Of course it was difficult being with you during your mood swings. We struggled with it, and you resented me. When you'd question me with neon-bright emotional colors, the chances were high that your answer would be fortune-cookie style." By fortune-cookie style, he meant not the truth, but what I wanted to hear.

> When you'd question me with neon-bright emotional colors, the chances were high that your answer would be fortune-cookie style." By fortune-cookie style, Yuri meant not the truth, but what I wanted to hear.

"My answer is that any disorder is always superimposed on a personality," Yuri continued. "Nasty people with a mild case of flu can be hard to take. Nice people are loved even when they have a debilitating illness. So, your illness has been less of a problem. You are free of malice. Our problems arose because of your tendency to manipulate, and I am particularly sensitive to any strong guiding hand. Still, I know that this is regarded as symptomatic of bipolar disorder. Manic-depressive illness not only presents a major challenge for those 'blessed' with it, but also for those of us around.

"Friendship presumes respect, not just flattering words and empty comforting. But you couldn't accept it when I gave it to you straight. You got mad and I froze, retreating into my comfortable shell. But even the Berlin Wall has come down, so let's not reconstruct any more fences! Remember the dear past, and let's not risk another fight. We've come back to friendship."

Marty: Embracing Loss and Making Adjustments

The most important person in my life is my husband, Marty. "I'm very proud of you," Marty said recently. "I'm excited you're doing so well, and I know you're happy when you're writing. But I regret not spending much time together anymore. You're always working."

> When I can't turn you off, I go into "overload." I tune out and don't hear anymore. It's very frustrating. Sometimes you'll ask me for an opinion, but you don't wait to hear my answer and you do what you want anyway.
>
> —MARTY ROSENFELD

I know that living with me is not easy for Marty. If our marriage were not so strong, there have been many times over the years that it could have collapsed. It's difficult for him to relate to my passion. He doesn't understand that a writing task can't be put down as easily as an accounting problem. But many writers share my intensity toward writing. It may be less about my bipolar disorder, and more about the nature of writing.

The mania that surfaces during my periods of intense writing exacerbates my bipolar condition, however. It is especially challenging for Marty during these episodes.

"When I walk in the door from work, you are still in your office," said Marty. "You're either at the computer or on the telephone. We eat dinner late. Afterwards, you fall asleep or go back to work. You're obsessed with work. Your work continues for hours, days, weeks, months, even years. It never stops. When you're not working, you talk about it, sometimes to the exclusion of everyone else in the room. You get so wrapped up in what you're saying that you lose sight of others wanting to speak. You eat, drink, and breathe your work, and you seldom quit before you're ready to collapse.

"When I can't turn you off, I go into 'overload.' I tune out and don't hear anymore. It's very frustrating. Sometimes you'll ask me for an opinion, but you don't wait to hear my answer and you do what you want anyway. You seem to pay more attention to other people than me."

It is clear that Marty experiences real stress and loneliness. His loss is real, and he longs to return to the earlier years of our marriage when life was much simpler. The adjustment for him has been twofold: dealing with the pain from all the stress I've put him through and the loneliness created by my absence.

Bernie: Empathic Without Feeling Threatened

Bernie instantly observed the mania in me at our initial meeting when I approached him about coauthoring this book. "I had eagerly looked forward to the meeting because I am attracted to people who exhibit excitement, energy, drive, and a certain lack of inhibition," said Bernie "This affinity is part of my personality as well as a driving force behind my work with clients. I have experienced this positive feeling when observing people, both in personal relationships and in clinical settings, who evidence certain manic qualities. But I remained somewhat apprehensive about our getting together. In part, this concern was related to the daunting diagnosis of bipolar illness.

"Some patients learn to manage their illness extremely well, but others are completely taken over by it. I had a history of experience to fuel my apprehension.

"Although my real fear was in not wanting to maintain a clinical lens during our meeting, I didn't want to be swept away in the whirlwind of excitement that I know such energy can elicit from me. At the same time, I admit to having been more than a little excited after learning about your two successfully published books. Both personally and professionally, this reassured me of your ability to channel your energy constructively."

Our scheduled one-hour meeting lasted two hours because both of us were engrossed. "You exuded so much energy," recalled Bernie, "and when you spoke, there was a sparkle in your eye as you communicated a clear passion about life and the desire for further enrichment. You demonstrated some expansiveness in gestures and were emotionally open."

When I described my book proposal and discussed past endeavors, Bernie recalled my exhibiting "great animation." He said, "As we shared, I experienced an internal dialogue which reflected my reactions to you and the surfacing of my personal issues regarding bipolar disorder."

Bernie found himself wondering if he would be able to keep up with me and meet our deadlines, especially when I boasted about getting by on a mere four hours of sleep for extended periods of time. He also wondered to what degree my potential for depressive or manic symptoms might interfere with and/or foster the progress of our joint project. Additionally, might he from time-to-time be persuaded against his better judgment to agree when he preferred to disagree?

"Gradually," said Bernie, "as the focus of our conversation shifted from professional to personal, I sensed a mutual understanding and genuine connection between us. We both knew intuitively that we were well-matched and could complement each other in a one-to-one relationship."

Bernie recognized me as someone who had transformed a negative condition into a positive and meaningful life. He recognized my energy, drive, and lack of inhibition; and, appropriately, he paused. Might he be swept away in the "whirlwind of excitement" that he knew such energy could create? Should apply the brakes? "I realized that it is at this junction that most of the turmoil arises for those who live with people with bipolar illness," said Bernie. "I stayed in this place for a moment, clarified my sensitivities and how I would address them, and I moved on."

Bernie found a lot of correlation between his reactions and those of the other people I asked about their experience of me as a person with bipolar disorder. He summed up what helps people who have a relationship with someone afflicted with this illness, "It is important that you know yourself, that you recognize the nature of manic and depressive symptoms, and that you are able to understand and recognize the interplay of these two polarized patterns of behavior."

SUMMARY

Throughout this chapter, we have identified how individuals are impacted in relationships with those who have bipolar illness. We have shared personal examples and highlighted several key issues to help shed light on the nature of such relationships. We emphasize that while many of the challenges inherent in such bonds parallel those of any two individuals developing a relationship, bipolar illness may more severely affect such intimacy at all levels.

> *Equally important to remember is that any disorder, as stated by Nancy's friend Yuri, is always superimposed on a personality; an individual with bipolar disorder still has a core personality throughout all phases of the illness.*

Equally important to remember is that any disorder, as stated by Nancy's friend Yuri, is always superimposed on a personality; an individual with bipolar disorder still has a core personality throughout all phases of the illness. One's core personality is always present, and that personality has a history of values, attitudes, interests, and ways of being even though it is colored by depression or mania. This is true for both people in the relationship.

Those who responded to Nancy's request for feedback all refer to issues of personality and the influence of bipolar illness. The issues, however, are often difficult to separate. Nancy's friend Lois clearly focuses on personality in her statement, "What I admire most is your willingness to accept criticism. You look for honesty in relationships." In contrast, Nancy alludes to the influence of bipolar illness, "If I happen to be at the height of a manic episode, [Lois] may defer saying something to me [until] she feels that I'm in a good place to listen."

It is human nature to construct a defining personality that includes the internal standards by which we assess how to think, feel, and behave Similarly, we construct a defining image of those with whom we form relationships. We may develop expectations about how they "should" behave in general, as well as how they "should" respond to our expectations. When someone appears to move beyond those parameters that we have defined as her "personality," we may be quick to say "it's not her." This is an inherent part of all relationships.

The impact of bipolar illness, however, challenges expectations and causes tension for both partners. It is this tension that leads to discussion or efforts to withdraw. Adding to this challenge is that any discussion becomes less meaningful or productive when symptoms are exacerbated. Each partner may feel less understood and experience the other as insensitive. How one responds to this tension is an individual decision based on one's personality, one's expectations of the relationship, the level of intimacy, and the commitment.

Living with someone who is afflicted with bipolar disorder presents challenges that are both similar to and yet different from other relationships. It is only by being aware of how our individual relationships are influenced by the illness that we can make them more fulfilling. When we possess such awareness, we are more able to experience our relationship as one with an individual who has bipolar illness rather than as a relationship with a bipolar person. In this way, we can still feel connected and maintain both empathy and compassion.

CHAPTER 12

Support Groups

THE VALUE OF a support group is the mutually helpful relationship that grows out of it—by helping others, you help yourself. These new friends, your fellow group members, can become your mainstay of support because you share something with everyone present: You all live with bipolar disorder. Your group becomes a forum for mutual acceptance, understanding, and self-discovery. A sense of camaraderie quickly develops among you.

Spending an evening with a group of strangers, all of whom have some type of mood disorder, may, at first, seem rather daunting. But as you become involved in discussion, you will feel buoyed by your new bond of support. Whereas you might have arrived feeling inherently defective (as people with any chronic illness often feel), by the time you leave you should feel improved. In the group, you have an opportunity to reach out to others and, in turn, to accept their help. You will no longer feel alone with your problems; others have been there, too.

"Dealing Effectively with Depression and Manic-Depression," a brochure offered by the National Depressive and Manic-Depressive Association (National DMDA), lists guidelines that form the foundation of effective recovery. Support groups throughout the country use the brochure. Here are the guidelines:

Hope With good symptom management, it is possible to experience long periods of wellness.

Personal Responsibility It is up to you, with the assistance of others, to take action to keep your moods stabilized.

Self-Advocacy Become an effective advocate for yourself so you can access the services and treatment you need and make the life you want for yourself.

Education Learn all that you can about depression and manic-depression. This allows you to make good decisions about all aspects of your treatment and life.

Support While working toward your wellness is up to you, the support of others is essential to maintaining your stability and enhancing the quality of your life.

PORTRAIT OF SUPPORT

The 1999 Annual Conference of National DMDA was in full swing, and its first group support sessions were under way. Nancy's support group had already begun by the time she entered the room. The leader was focusing on colors and seasonal changes as good indicators of mood fluctuations.

"When I glanced around the room, I instantly became aware of the group's somber mood," said Nancy. "Most attendees appeared to be mildly to severely depressed."

"Autumn is the worst time of year for me," said one woman. "I think of death. I don't want to leave the house. I can't sleep at night."

"I agree," said another woman. "Autumn means that winter is just around the corner. I go into a deep depression every January. It's so cold and gloomy."

"Bright summer days are most disturbing to me," added a young man who appeared to be in his mid-to-late twenties. "I avoid the sunshine. Everyone's cheer makes me feel worse."

"I know what you mean," responded a young woman of about the same age. She was dressed in black. "I feel the same way about holidays. Nothing depresses me more than that time between Thanksgiving and New Year's Day. The colored lights, matched by everyone's happy faces, set me off. I want to pull the covers over my head and not wake up until the season's over."

"I find summer days depressing," said another young woman. "But I take prescription medication and the drugs work for me. I'm also outgoing and active; I exercise regularly and date often. I don't need [psychological] therapy, but I do attend AA [Alcohol Anonymous]. I would like to reach the point when *nothing* bothers me."

"How boring," somebody commented.

"We'll get there, but not until we're dead," declared another.

> Their comments were not meant to be critical, but they were demonstrating a type of reality check that participants must learn to do on their own in managing their illness.

The comments of the members of this support group illustrate the impact that a session can have on those in attendance. Their comments were not meant to be critical, but they were demonstrating a type of reality check that participants must learn to do on their own in managing their illness.

Members are encouraged to express their thoughts freely and not hold back. Support groups offer a safe haven. The young woman who found summers depressing had done a reality check and was honest about her "weakness." By taking positive steps to combat her problems, she positioned herself to control her own disorder. She also projected into the future by striving to meet a goal. Modeling the skills needed to cope with living with bipolar disorder is one of the ways in which a support group can be most valuable.

The discussion turned to the significance of color.

"I don't wear bright colors because I don't want to stand out," said a middle-aged woman who was clad from head to toe in black. "If I wear black and sit in the back of the room, nobody will notice me; and I won't be called on to participate. Black makes me feel safe."

Somebody mentioned "hospital white," and a woman blurted out, "White is cheap and sterile and reminds me of death and dying, so why dress that way?" She came decked out in a flashy, colorful costume.

In a setting where people are free to express their feelings without fear of recrimination, they can be helped to rid themselves of old patterns of thinking. Many of us were brought up to believe that healthy, well-adjusted people are those who cope independently with the pressures and demands of life. For example: men aren't supposed to cry, it's a sign of weakness; and, we shouldn't burden others with our troubles because everyone has problems of their own. Misconceptions such as these provide good topics for support groups. Members listen attentively to each other and provide necessary feedback. Group leaders are trained to skillfully direct such discussions so participants will receive maximum benefit.

At the same conference, Dr. Drew Pinsky, commonly referred to as "Dr. Drew," moderated a panel discussion on "Intimacy and Depression." The setting was a large conference hall with approximately two hundred attendees. Seated in front on a raised platform was Dr. Drew, cohost of *Loveline*, the nationally syndicated radio and MTV call-in show, and a panel of four that had been assembled to educate individuals and couples on how to cope with the debilitating effect depression can have on relationships. The first two panelists were a husband-and-wife team—she, a doctor of psychology; he, a licensed psychiatric social worker. Even they, two professionals, reported being affected by public stigma after the wife's diagnosis with clinical depression. Their good fortune was their base of support—the strong foundation of a 20-year marriage.

"As therapists, you'd think we would have been better prepared to deal with the reality of my wife's hospitalization," the man told the audience gathered for the panel. "But that was not the case. Immediately following her admittance, we told people that she had entered the hospital because of 'extreme exhaustion.' I doubt anyone was fooled by that explanation. Yet public stigma colored our attitudes, too."

"I had wished for a quick fix," said his wife, "but realistically I knew there were no instant cures. Drug therapy for deep clinical depression takes anywhere from three to six weeks and has a 70-percent chance of being effective. I also had a 70-percent chance of suffering some loss of my natural sex drive. Depression leaves patients feeling sexless."

The following are some of the questions the audience asked Dr. Drew.

"I live with bipolar, and my first marriage was wrecked because of my infidelity," said one man in the audience. "I've since remarried and I want to preserve that relationship, but I'm very worried because the same feelings that destroyed my first marriage are returning. What can I do?"

"You might benefit from couples therapy," suggested Dr. Drew. "Those rumblings you describe may also be symptomatic of mania. Perhaps a mood stabilizer such as lithium might help."

A 25-year-old man stated that he was fearful of intimacy, and said, "I've been on lithium for 15 years. Every time I become attracted to a woman I have a manic attack."

"Your attraction to women may cause mood escalation. I'd advise talking to your doctor about reevaluating the dosage of your medication," Dr. Drew responded.

A female audience member spoke up, "In a dating situation, when is it appropriate to discuss my bipolar condition?"

"A normal process of self-disclosure generally develops in any serious dating relationship. You'll know when you have established a level of trust," advised Dr. Drew.

"Since I began taking mood stabilizers to control my bipolar illness, I can no longer achieve orgasm. What steps can be taken to get back lust?" another woman asked.

"This is a step-by-step process. It begins with enjoyment, then warmth, companionship, and sensitivity until, finally, that craving for love and lust reemerges," Dr. Drew explained.

Later in the day, another conference support group focused on the stigma of mental illness. "It takes courage to be yourself and face up to stigma," the group leader said.

"But nobody understands our internal agony," someone shouted. "People with bipolar illness are unfairly prejudged."

"I've been depressed since birth," offered a woman participant. She sat hunched over in her chair, disheveled and red-eyed. "I've had many suicidal thoughts. But people don't want to know about it. Nobody is interested; they're like dead, won't acknowledge anything."

"It's true that many folks don't understand," replied the leader. "But this is what National DMDA is all about. We must educate the public so people *will* understand and help us."

A man who referred to himself as "the mad rocket scientist," said, "Not long ago I was written up at work for being 'confrontational' during a manic episode. Although I knew I was off the wall, I couldn't help myself. I hope that lithium will answer my needs because another episode like this may cost me my job."

Sitting adjacent to the mad rocket scientist was a former psychiatric social worker who was now on disability. "Bipolar illness offers us an exquisite ability to project outwardly a strong persona, an image much more powerful than we may actually feel internally," she commented. Meanwhile, the group leader listened and, from time-to-time, offered some helpful advice. Mostly, however, the leader positioned herself to let the discussion flow freely and be guided by its participants.

"What about health insurance companies?" inquired the leader. "Don't most insurance agents prey on stigma and on our feelings of shame and discomfort?"

A former executive from a large corporation responded, "Unfortunately, that's exactly how the mental health system works in New

York. I was way up there on the corporate ladder, but I faced lots of stigma. I did the best I could, but I soon saw the writing on the wall and knew that it was time to quit. I had no more energy to fight, and then I became desperately depressed. Now I can talk about the stigma that I faced."

"I've lost lots of jobs and relationships," someone echoed. "But once I realized that stigma was self-projected, I was able to cast it aside."

Across the room from Nancy sat a tall, handsome man with an athletic build who appeared to be no older than his early forties. He introduced himself as from Dallas, Texas. Seemingly self-assured and with a quick smile he began.

"Eight days ago I was diagnosed with manic-depressive illness," he said. "'Shit,' I told my buddies that day! 'I'm bipolar.'" Everyone in the room fell silent. "I got depressed," he continued. "I had some fleeting suicidal thoughts, and then got drunk. I only sobered up a couple days ago."

The room had gone quiet as he spoke. After a few moments pause, a woman said, "I used to work on a hospital psychiatric ward. But now, my 'normal' friends think this [her illness] is a *hobby*." This woman was referring to the "accepted" opinion that was held by a group of uninformed friends. They had mistakenly interpreted what appeared to them as their friend's "melodramatic" pattern of behavior.

Finally, all tension broke loose as the room swelled with laughter. As depression is contagious, so is humor. Laughter is far removed from a depressed state and, therefore, can be very therapeutic.

When the laughter had subsided, Nancy spoke: "I was diagnosed with bipolar disorder several years ago. My condition is genetic, but was triggered by a sudden shock. I plummeted to Hell from the top of Mount Everest. What ultimately saved me was my ability to write. Writing is cathartic, and that's very therapeutic. For me it was better medicine than any form of therapy, either drug or psychological. I do take daily antidepressants, though." She added, "Nobody on Earth escapes life without some form of disability. For better or worse, most of us here were dealt bipolar disorder. Others survive even greater disabilities. I prefer to regard bipolar disorder as a 'gift.' I do my best creative writing in a hypomanic state. By looking at the positive side of bipolar disorder, for me it no longer carries a stigma. In a very real sense, my life has been enriched as a result of my condition."

The last to respond to the group leader's focus on stigma was a professor of veterinary medicine who was up for tenure. Her immediate supervisor had recently cautioned her not to disclose the nature of her illness for fear of what "others might think." Despite the apparent stigma, this soon-to-be-tenured professor echoed Nancy's belief when she stated, "Bipolar *is* a gift. I'll wear it well."

> Nobody on Earth escapes life without some form of disability. For better or worse, most of us here were dealt bipolar disorder. Others survive even greater disabilities. I prefer to regard bipolar disorder as a "gift."
>
> —NANCY ROSENFELD

Support groups promote closeness, a result of participants' opening up to each other and sharing both deep pleasures and profound pain. Members learn to trust one another. All group discussions remain confidential, and advice from fellow participants is taken seriously inasmuch as everyone present has "been there" (to Hell and back), at least once.

Support groups are a major function of National DMDA. These groups have medical advisers, but are wholly run and operated by patients or family members. Some of the chapters even have a lending library, newsletter, fundraisers, and other organized activities. Group leaders and participants maintain contact with the national organization and, vis-a-vis, the organization keeps tabs on them. Become a member! For more information on how and where to find a support group in your area, see the appendix, "Resources for Information."

Appendix: Resources for Information

American Association for Geriatric
  Psychiatry
7910 Woodmont Avenue,
  Suite 11050
Bethesda, MD 20815
Phone: (301) 654-7850
Web site: www.aagpgpa.org

American Association for Marriage
  and Family Therapy
1133 15th Street, Northwest,
  Suite 300
Washington, DC 20005
Phone: (202) 452-0109
Web site: www.aamft.org

American Association of Child
  and Adolescent Psychiatry
3615 Wisconsin Avenue, Northwest
Washington, DC 20016
Phone: (202) 966-7300
Web site: www.aacap.org

American Association of
  Suicidology
4201 Connecticut Avenue,
  Northwest, Suite 408
Washington, DC 20008
Phone: (202) 237-2280

Fax: (202) 237-2282
Web site: www.suicidology.org

American Foundation for Suicide
  Prevention
120 Wall Street, 22nd Floor
New York, NY 10005
Phone: (888) 333-2377
Fax: (212) 363-6237
Web site: www.afsp.org

American Psychiatric Association
1400 K Street, Northwest
Washington, DC 20005
Phone: (888) 357-7924
Web site: www.psych.org

American Psychological Association
750 First Street, Northeast
Washington, DC 20002
Phone: (202) 336-5700 or
  (800) 374-3120
Web site: www.apa.org

Anxiety Disorders Association
  of America
11900 Parklawn Drive, Suite 100
Rockville, MD 20852
Phone: (301) 231-9350
Fax: (301) 231-7392
Web site: www.adaa.org

Bazelon Center
1101 15th Street, Northwest,
    Suite 1212
Washington, DC 20005
Phone: (202) 467-5730
Web site: www.bazelon.org

Bipolar Disorders Portal:
    Your Gateway to the Web
Web site: www.pendulum.org

BPSO Public Pages
Web site: www.bpso.org

Centers for Disease Control
    and Prevention
National Center for Injury
    Prevention and Control
Web site: www.cdc.gov/ncipc

Child and Adolescent
    Bipolar Foundation
Web site: www.cabf.org

Depression After Delivery
P.O. Box 1282
Morrisville, PA 19607
Phone: (800) 944-4773
Web site: www.infotrail.com
    /dad/dad.html

Depression and Related
    Affective Disorders Association
The John Hopkins Hospital,
    Meyer 3-181
600 North Wolfe Street
Baltimore, MD 21287
Phone: (410) 955-4647
Fax: (410) 614-3241
Web site: www.med.jhu.edu
    /drada

Health Resources and Services
    Administration
Web site: www.hrsa.dhhs.gov

Men's Health Network
P.O. Box 75972
Washington, DC 20013
Phone: (888) MEN-2-MEN
Web site: www.info@
    menshealthnetwork.org

National Alliance for Research on
    Schizophrenia and Depression
60 Cutter Mill Road, Suite 404
Great Neck, NY 11021
Phone: (516) 829-0091
Fax: (516) 487-6930
Web site: www.narsad.org

National Alliance for the
    Mentally Ill
2107 Wilson Boulevard, Suite 300
Arlington, VA 22201
Phone: (703) 524-7600 or
    (800) 950-6264
Fax: (703) 524-9094
Web site: www.nami.org

National Association of Social
    Workers
750 First Street, Northeast,
    Suite 700
Washington, DC 20002
Phone: (800) 638-8799
Web site: www.socialworkers.org

National Depressive and
    Manic-Depressive Association
730 North Franklin Street,
    Suite 501

Chicago, IL 60610
Phone: (800) 826-3632
Fax: (312) 642-7243
Web site: www.ndmda.org

National Foundation for
  Depressive Illness
P.O. Box 2257
New York, NY 10116
Phone: (800) 239-1265
Web site: www.depression.org

National Institute of Mental Health
6001 Executive Boulevard
Bethesda, MD 20892
Phone: (800) 421-4211
Web site: www.nimh.nih.gov

National Institute of Mental Health
  Suicide Research Consortium
Web site:www.nimh.nih.gov
  /research/suicide.htm

National Institute on Alcohol
  Abuse and Alcoholism
6000 Executive Boulevard,
  Willco Building
Bethesda, MD 20892
Web site: www.niaaa.nih.gov

National Institute on Drug Abuse
6001 Executive Boulevard
Bethesda, MD 20892
Phone: (800) 644-6432
Web site: www.nida.nih.gov

National Mental Health
  Association
1201 Prince Street
Alexandria, VA 22314
Phone: (800) 969-6642

Fax: (703) 684-5968
Web site: www.nmha.org

National Women's Health Resource
  Center
120 Albany Street, Suite 820
New Brunswick, NJ 08901
Phone: (877) 986-9472 or
  (732) 828-8575
Web site: www.healthywomen.org

Obsessive-Compulsive Foundation
337 Notch Hill Road
North Branford, CT 06471
Phone: (203) 315-2190
Web site: www.ocfoundation.org

RnetHealth.com, Inc.
506 Santa Monica Boulevard,
  Suite 400
Santa Monica, California 90401
Phone: (310) 393-3979
Fax: (310) 393-5749
Web site: www.mymind
  andbody.com

Screening for Mental Health, Inc.
One Washington Street, Suite 304
Wellesley Hills, MA 02481
Phone: (800) 573-4433
  (Depression Screening)
Fax: (781) 431-7447
Web site: www.nmisp.org

Sexual Function Health Council
American Foundation for Urologic
  Disease
300 West Pratt Street, Suite 401
Baltimore, MD 21201
Phone: (800) 242-2383
Web site: www.afud.org

Substance Abuse and
   Mental Health Services
Web site: www.samhsa.gov

Suicide Prevention
   Advocacy Network
5034 Odin's Way
Marietta, GA 30068
Phone: (888) 649-1366
Fax: (770) 642-1419
Web site: www.spanusa.org

Support Group.com
   Home Page
Web site: www.support-group.com
   /index.htm

Surgeon General of the
   United States
Web site: www.surgeongeneral.gov

Notes

CHAPTER 1

1. Deborah Bullwinkel is the former program director of the National Depressive Manic-Depressive Association (National DMDA), the National organization that was cofounded by Jan Fawcett, M.D.

2. Sol Wachtler, *After the Madness: A Judge's Own Prison Memoir*, New York: Random House, 1997.

3. www.s-t.com/daily/01-98/01-05-98/c01ae100.htm.

4. Kathy Cronkite, *On the Edge of Darkness*, New York: Delta, 1995.

5. Ibid.

6. www.s-t.com/daily/01-98/01-05-98/c01ae100.htm.

7. Ibid.

8. Ibid.

9. Kathy Cronkite, *On the Edge of Darkness*, New York: Delta, 1995.

10. Ibid.

11. Ibid.

12. Ibid.

13. Kay Redfield Jamison, *An Unquiet Mind*, New York: Vintage Books, 1996.

14. Kathy Cronkite, *On the Edge of Darkness*, New York: Delta, 1995.

15. Frederick K. Goodwin, M.D., and Kay Redfield Jamison, Ph.D., *Manic-Depressive Illness*, New York: Oxford University Press, 1990.

16. Kay Redfield Jamison, *Night Falls Fast*, New York: Alfred A. Knopf, 1999.

17. Frederick K. Goodwin, M.D., and Kay Redfield Jamison, Ph.D., *Manic-Depressive Illness*, New York: Oxford University Press, 1990.

18. Ibid.

19. "What It Would Really Take," *Time*, June 17, 1999, pp 54–55.

20. "Depression Confession," *The Nation*, June 28, 1999, p. 10.

21. "Tipper Gore and Rosalynn Carter on America's Mental Health Crisis," *Psychology Today*, September/October, 1999, p. 31.

22. "What It Would Really Take," *Time*, June 17, 1999, pp 54–55.

CHAPTER 2

1. Frederick K. Goodwin, M.D., and Kay Redfield Jamison, Ph.D., *Manic-Depressive Illness*, New York: Oxford University Press, 1990.

2. Demitri Papolos, M.D., and Janice Papolos, *Overcoming Depression*, NewYork: HarperPerennial, 1997.

3. Frederick K. Goodwin, M.D., and Kay Redfield Jamison, Ph.D., *Manic-Depressive Illness*, New York: Oxford University Press, 1990.

4. Ibid.

CHAPTER 3

1. Lewis A. Opler, M.D., Ph.D., and Carol Bialkowski, *Prozac and Other Psychiatric Drugs: Everything You Need to Know*, New York: Pocket Books, 1996.

2. Gershon, Elliot S. and colleagues, summarized from A. Bertelsen: A Danish twin study of manic-depressive disorders; M. Schou, E. Strömgren, eds: Origin, Prevention and Treatmentof Affective Disorders. London: Academic Press, 1979; pp 227–239 in Frederick K. Goodwin, M.D., and Kay Redfield Jamison, Ph.D., *Manic-Depressive Illness*, New York: Oxford University Press, 1990.

3. *Tidsskr Nor Laegeforen*; 1999, September 20; 119, (22):3322–8.

4. Samuel H. Barondes, introduction to the "Report of the NIMH Genetics Workgroup," *Biological Psychiatry*, March 1,1999; 45; 559–602).

5. Ibid.

6. Steven H. Hyman, M.D., "Introduction to the Complex Genetics of Mental Disorders," *Biological Psychiatry*, March 1, 1999; vol 45: no 5; 518–521.

7. Murray, C.J., Lopez, A.D. "Global Mortality, Disability, and the Contribution of Risk Factors: Global Burden of Disease Study," *The Lancet*; May 17, 1997; 349 (9063):1436–42.

8. Gershon, Elliot S. and colleagues, summarized from A. Bertelsen: A Danish twin study of manic-depressive disorders; M. Schou, E. Strömgren, eds: Origin, Prevention and Treatment of Affective Disorders. London: Academic Press, 1979; pp 227-239 in Frederick K. Goodwin, M.D., and Kay Redfield Jamison, Ph.D., *Manic-Depressive Illness*, New York: Oxford University Press, 1990.

9. Manji, H.K., Moore,GJ, Cheng J. J, *Clinical Psychiatry*, 2000; 61 suppl; 9:82–96.

10. Sapolsky, Dr. Robert; *Nature Neuroscience*; March 2000; "Enrichment induces structural changes and recovery

from non-spatial memory deficits in CA1-NMDART-knockout mice"; commenting on the study of Ramponc, J.Z. Tsien, and Associates; Princeton University.

CHAPTER 4

1. National Depressive and Manic-Depressive Association, "Consensus Statement on the Undertreatment of Depression," *Journal of the American Medical Association* 277:4 (January 22/29, 1997).

2. L. Tondo and R.J. Baldessarini, "Reduced Suicide Risk During Lithium Maintenance Treatment," *Journal of Clinical Psychiatry*, 61 (2000) Supplement 9:97–104.

3. Lewis A. Opler, M.D., Ph.D., and Carol Bialkowski, *Prozac and Other Psychiatric Drugs: Everything You Need to Know*, New York: Pocket Books, 1996.

4. Steven Bratman, M.D., *Beat Depression with St. John's Wort*, Roseville, CA: Prima Publishing, 1997.

5. Jerrold F. Rosenbaum, M.D., and Steffany Fredman, "Medication Controversies in the Treatment of Bipolar Disorder," and Frederick K. Goodwin, M.D., and Tracey L. Irvin, M.D., "General Guidelines and Intricacies in the Treatment of Bipolar Disorder," both from the 1999 American Psychiatric Association Annual Meeting; www.medscape.com.

6. 1999 online survey, National Depressive and Manic-Depressive Association.

CHAPTER 5

1. D. Burns, *Feeling Good: Ten Days to Self-Esteem*, New York: Avon, 1992.

2. A. Beck, B. Shaw, and G. Emery, *Cognitive Therapy of Depression*, New York: Guilford Press, 1979.

3. Ibid.

4. Ibid.

5. Ibid.

6. D. Burns, *Feeling Good: The New Mood Therapy*, New York: Avon, 1992.

7. Ibid.

8. A. Weissman, "The Dysfunctional Attitudes Scale: A Validation Study," *Dissertation Abstracts International*, 40 (1979): 1389–1390.

9. Kay Redfield Jamison, *An Unquiet Mind*, New York: Vintage Books, 1996.

10. K. Dobson, *The Handbook of Cognitive Behavioral Therapies*, New York: Guilford Press, 1988.

11. T. D'Zurilla and M. Goldfried, "Problem Solving and Behavior Modification," *Journal of Abnormal Psychology*, vol 78, 1971. (in K. Dobson)

12. M. Goldfried and G. Davison, *Clinical Behavior Therapy*, New York: Holt, Rinehart and Winston, 1976.

13. R. Lazarus and S. Folman, *Stress, Appraisal and Coping*, New York: Springer, 1984.

14. K. Dobson, *The Handbook of Cognitive Behavioral Therapies*, New York: Guilford Press, 1988.

CHAPTER 6

1. Richard C.W. Hall, M.D., Dennis E. Platt, M.D., and Ryan C.W. Hall, "Suicide Risk Assessment: A Review of Risk Factors for Suicide in 100 Patients Who Made Severe Suicide Attempts," *Psychosomatics*, 40 (February 1999): 18–27.

2. Ibid.

3. Danielle Steel, *His Bright Light*, New York: Delacorte Press, 1998.

4. In 1978, Jan Fawcett participated as a principal investigator in a 15-year collaborative study of suicide, National Institute of Mental Health. The study is still in progress. Results of this

study were published in *American Journal of Psychiatry*, 147 (1990): 1189–1194.

5. Eli Robins, *The Final Months*, New York: Oxford University Press, 1981.

6. R.W. Ettlinger and P. Flordh, "Attempted Suicide: Experience of 500 Cases at a General Hospital," *ACTA Psychiatrica Nerol Scan;* 1955; 103 (suppl):1–45.

7. M.C. Tejedor, A. Diaz, J.J. Castillon, J.M. Pericay, "Attempted Suicide: Repetition and Survival—Findings of a Follow-up Study," *ACTA Psychiatr Scand*, September 1999; 100; 3: 205–211.

8. A. Roy, G. Rylander, M. Sachiapone, "Genetics of Suicide. Family Studies and Molecular Genetics," *Annals of New York Academy of Sciences*, December 1997; 29; 836: 135–57.

9. Jan Fawcett, W.A. Scheftner, L. Fogg, D.C. Clark, M.A. Young, D. Hedeker, and R. Gibbons. "Time-Related Predictors of Suicide in Major Affective Disorder," *American Journal of Psychiatry*, 147 (1990): 1189–1194.

10. Ibid.

11. Kay Redfield Jamison, *Night Falls Fast*, New York: Alfred A. Knopf, 1999.

12. Michael Burlingame, *The Inner World of Abraham Lincoln*, Champagne, IL: University of Illinois Press, 1994.

13. Richard C.W. Hall, M.D., Dennis E. Platt, M.D., and Ryan C.W. Hall, "Suicide Risk Assessment: A Review of Risk Factors for Suicide in 100 Patients Who Made Severe Suicide Attempts," *Psychosomatics*, 40 (February 1999): 18–27.

CHAPTER 7

1. Paul Fink and Allan Tasman, *Stigma and Mental Illness*, Washington, D.C.: American Psychiatric Press, 1992.

2. Richard Chessick, *Intensive Psychotherapy*, New York: Jason Aronson, 1974.

3. E. Dodds, *The Greeks and the Irrational*, Boston: Beacon Press, 1957 in P. Fink and A. Tasman, 1992.

4. Paul Fink and Allan Tasman, *Stigma and Mental Illness*, Washington, D.C.: American Psychiatric Press, 1992.

5. Michael Lewis, *Shame: The Exposed Self*, New York: Free Press, 1995.

6. Ibid.

7. Kathy Cronkite, *On the Edge of Darkness*, New York: Delta, 1995.

8. Ibid.

9. Ibid.

10. Ibid.

11. Michael Lewis, *Shame: The Exposed Self*, New York: Free Press, 1995.

12. Martin Seligman, *Learned Optimism*, New York: Pocket Books, 1998.

13. Michael Lewis, *Shame: The Exposed Self*, New York: Pocket Books, 1998.

14. Susan Sontag, *Illness As Metaphor and AIDS and Its Metaphors*, New York: Peter Smith Publishing, 1995.

15. Ibid.

16. Ibid.

17. Harold S. Kushner, *How Good Do We Have to Be?*, New York: Little, Brown and Company, 1997.

18. Irvin Esters, et al., "Effects of a Unit of Instruction in Mental Health on Rural Adolescents' Conceptions of Mental Illness and Attitudes about Seeking Help," *Adolescence*, 33:130 (Summer 1998): 469–476.

19. Kathryn Foxhall, "APA is key to anti-stigma campaign," *Monitor on Psychology*, Vol 31, No 7, July/August, 48-49, 2000.

CHAPTER 8

1. Martin E. P. Seligman, *Learned Optimism*, New York: Pocket Books, 1998.

2. Rollo May, *Existence*, New York: Basic Books, 1958.

3. Ibid.

4. Kay Redfield Jamison, *Touched with Fire*, New York: Free Press, 1994.

5. Ibid.

6. Shelley E. Taylor, *Positive Illusions*, New York: Basic Books, 1989.

7. Kay Redfield Jamison, *An Unquiet Mind*, New York: Vintage, 1995.

8. Mihaly Csikszentmihalyi, *Flow: The Psychology of Optimal Experience*, New York: HarperPerennial, 1991.

9. Ibid.

10. Kay Redfield Jamison, *An Unquiet Mind*, New York: Vintage, 1995.

11. Ibid.

12. Martin E. P. Seligman, *Learned Optimism*, New York: Pocket Books, 1998.

13. Daniel Goleman, *Emotional Intelligence*, New York: Bantam Books, 1995.

CHAPTER 9

1. Victor E. Frankl, *Man's Search for Ultimate Meaning*, New York: Insight Books, 1997.

2. Artemis P. Simopoulos, M.D., and Jo Robinson, *The Omega Plan*, New York: HarperCollins, 1998.

3. Ibid.

4. Susan Musikanth, *Stress Matters*, Johannesburg, South Africa: William Waterman, 1996.

5. Susan Musikanth, *Depression Matters*, Johannesburg, South Africa: Delta Books, 1997.

6. Mary Ellen Copeland, M.S., *Living Without Depression and Manic-Depression*, Oakland, CA: New Harbinger, 1994.

7. Ada P. Kahn, M.P.H., and Sheila Kimmel, M.A., *Empower Yourself: Every Woman's Guide to Self-Esteem*, New York: Avon Books, 1997.

8. Carl Jung, *The Undiscovered Self,* New York: Little, Brown and Company, 1957.

9. Mary Ellen Copeland, M.S., *Living Without Depression and Manic-Depression,* Oakland, CA: New Harbinger, 1994.

10. Ada P. Kahn, M.P.H., and Sheila Kimmel, M.A., *Empower Yourself: Every Woman's Guide to Self-Esteem,* New York: Avon Books, 1997.

11. J. Krishnamurti, *Freedom from the Known,* New York: HarperCollins, 1969.

CHAPTER 10

1. J. McClellan and J. Werry, "Practice Parameters for the Assessment and Treatment of Children and Adolescents with Bipolar Illness," *Journal of the American Academy of Child and Adolescent Psychiatry,* 36 (1997): 138–157.

2. M. Hellander, executive director, Child and Adolescent Bipolar Foundation, personal communication.

3. B. Geller and J. Luby, "Child and Adolescent Bipolar Disorder: A Review of the Past Ten Years," *Journal of the American Academy of Child and Adolescent Psychiatry,* 36 (1997): 1168–1176.

4. Ibid.

5. D. Papolos and J. Papolos, *The Bipolar Child,* New York: Broadway Books, 1999.

6. Kay Redfield Jamison, *Night Falls Fast,* New York: Alfred Knopf,1999, 48.

7. M. Strober, et al. "Recovery and Relapse in Adolescents with Bipolar Illness: A Five-Year Naturalistic Study," *American Journal of the Academy of Child and Adolescent Psychiatry,* 34 (1995): 724–731.

8. J. McClellan and J. Werry, "Practice Parameters for the Assessment and Treatment of Children and Adolescents with Bipolar Illness," *Journal of the American Academy of Child and Adolescent Psychiatry,* 36 (1997): 138–157.

9. American Psychiatric Association, *Diagnostic and Statistical Manual of Mental Disorders*, 4th ed., Washington, DC, 1994.

10. M. Bowring and M. Kovacs, "Difficulties in Diagnosing Manic Disorders in Children and Adolescents," *Journal of the American Academy of Child and Adolescent Psychiatry*, 31 (1992): 611–614.

11. F. Goodwin and K. Jamison, *Manic-Depressive Illness*, New York; Oxford University Press, 1990.

12. C. Sarnii, *The Development of Emotional Competence*, New York: The Guilford Press, 1999.

13. R. Gittelman, et al., "Hyperactive Boys Almost Grown Up," *Archives of General Psychiatry*, 42 (1985): 937–947.

14. J. Biederman et al., "Attention-Deficit Hyperactivity Disorder and Juvenile Mania: An Overlooked Comorbidity?" *Journal of the American Academy of Child and Adolescent Psychiatry*, 35 (1996):997–1008.

15. C. Popper, "Diagnosing Bipolar vs. ADHD: A Pharmacological Point of View," *The Link*, 13, 1996 in D. Papolos and J. Papolos, *The Bipolar Child*, New York: Broadway Books, 1999.

16. E. Costello, "Child Psychiatric Disorders and Their Correlates: A Primary Care Pediatric Sample," *Journal of the American Academy of Child and Adolescent Psychiatry*, 28 (1989): 851–855.

17. T. Achenbach, *The Child Behavior Checklist*, T. Achenbach, Publisher, 1980–94 in J. Impara and B. Plake, *The Thirteenth Mental Measurement Yearbook*, Lincoln, Nebraska: Buros Institute of Mental Measurements, 1998.

18. P.L. Hazell, et al., "Confirmation that the Child Behavior Checklist Clinical Scales Discriminate Juvenile Mania from Attention Deficit Hyperactivity Disorder," *Journal of Pediatric Child Health*, 35:2 (1999): 199–203.

19. M. Kovacs and M. Pollock, "Bipolar Disorder and Co-morbid Conduct Disorder in Childhood and Adolescence," *Journal of*

the American Academy of Child and Adolescent Psychiatry, 34 (1995): 715–723.

20. D. Papolos and J. Papolos, *The Bipolar Child*, New York: Broadway Books, 1999.

21. M. Strober, et al., "A Family Study of Bipolar I Disorder in Adolescence: Early Onset of Symptoms Linked to Increased Familial Loading and Lithium Resistance." *Journal of Affective Disorders*, 15 (1988): 255–268.

22. Grigoroiu-Serbanescu, et al., "Clinical evidence for genomic imprinting in bipolar I disorder," *ACTA Psychiatrica Scandinavica*, 92(5):365-70, 1995 Nov.

23. B. Geller and J. Luby, "Child and Adolescent Bipolar Disorder: A Review of the Past Ten Years," *Journal of the American Academy of Child and Adolescent Psychiatry*, 36 (1997): 1168–1176.

24. "Child and Adolescent Bipolar Disorder: An Update from the National Institute of Mental Health," (April 2000), Web site: and L. Tondo, "Antisuicidal Effect of Lithium Treatment in Major Mood Disorders," *The Harvard Medical School Guide to Suicide Assessment and Intervention*, D, Jacobs, ed., San Francisco: Jossey-Bass Publishers, 1998.

25. James Chandler, M.D., "Bipolar Affective Disorder (Manic Depressive Disorder) in Children and Adolescents," Web site: www.klis.com/chandler/pamphlet/bipolar/bipolarpamphlet.htm.

26. R. Baldessarini and J. Papolos, *The Bipolar Child*, New York: Broadway Books, 1999.

27. J. McClellan and J. Werry, "Practice Parameters for the Assessment and Treatment of Children and Adolescents with Bipolar Illness," *Journal of the American Academy of Child and Adolescent Psychiatry*, 36 (1997): 138–157.

28. D. Papolos and J. Papolos, *The Bipolar Child*, New York: Broadway Books, 1999.

CHAPTER 11

1. D.J. Miklowitz and J.M. Hooley, "Developing Family Psycho-educational Treatments for Patients with Bipolar and Other Severe Psychiatric Disorders: A Pathway from Basic Research to Clinical Trials," *Journal of Marital and Family Therapy*, 24 (1998): 419–435.
2. T.L. Simoneau and D.J. Miklowitz, "Expressed Emotion and Interactional Patterns in the Family of Bipolar Patients," *Journal of Abnormal Psychology*, 107 (1998): 497–507.

Glossary

amygdala   Almond-sized group of cells which assign positive or negative emotional responses to experience.

anhedonia   Loss of ability to feel pleasure.

basal ganglia   An area of the brain known to control body movement; may have an effect on emotional responses.

bipolar disorder   Formerly known as manic-depressive illness; a mood disorder characterized by at least one episode of mania or hypomania.

cerebral cortex   The right and left hemispheres of the brain.

clinical depression   Depressed mood, low energy, loss of capacity for pleasure, changes in sleep, appetite lasting more than two weeks and causing impairment of work or social function.

cingulate gyrus   Part of the limbic system, channels affect (emotions, feelings) and drive.

cognitive therapy   Psychotherapy focusing on identifying distortions of thinking and challenging and replacing them with more realistic thoughts.

concordant   When referring to diseases in twins, both members of the twin pair are affected.

congenital   Being born with, genetically or during development *in utero* prior to birth.

cyclothymia   The mildest form of bipolar disorder, including numerous periods of hypomania and mild depression.

dementia   Severe impairment or loss of intellectual capacity and personality integration.

discordant   When referring to diseases in twins, affecting only one twin.

dizygotic twins (DZ)   Fraternal twins.

dysthymia   Depressive neurosis.

ECT (electroconvulsive therapy)   Commonly known as "shock therapy," works by transmitting weak currents through the brain to cause seizure while patient is anesthetized.

electroencephalogram (EEG)   Measures electrical brain wave frequencies.

etiology   Concerning the cause, or root of, an illness.

hippocampus   Folded area of the base of the brain in the temporal lobes, controlling short-term memory and conversion to long-term memory which involve intellectual and emotional responses.

hyperthymia   *See* cyclothymia.

hypomania   A mild form of mania that neither causes psychosis nor leads to hospitalization.

hypothalamus   A cluster of nerve cells that controls appetite, sexual responses, mood responses, and the pituitary gland.

limbic system   Near center of brain, composed of amygdala, cingulate gyrus, hippocampus, hypothalamus, pituitary gland.

lithium   A mood stabilizing drug, used to treat the manic phase of bipolar disorder.

MAOI   *See* monoamine oxidase inhibitors.

manic depression   *See* bipolar disorder.

monoamine oxidase inhibitors   Tricyclic antidepressants.

monozygotic twins (MZ)   Identical twins.

MRI   Magnetic resonance imaging scans, which produce pictures of the body (including the brain) using magnetic fields and radio waves.

neurotransmitter   A biochemical substance released by nerve endings which chemically transmit nerve impulses.

neurotropic substances   Promote growth and repair of nerve tissue.

neutron   An electrically neutral atomic particle.

obsessive-compulsive disorder   Recurrent and intrusive thoughts and impulses (obsessions) and repetitive behaviors or mental acts (compulsions) causing discomfort that arises from anxiety/depression.

oligogenic inheritance   Inheritance due to several genes.

PET   Positron emission tomography (scans), a means of measuring brain metabolism.

pituitary gland   Major endocrine gland at base of brain, controls growth and regulates hormonal stress.

prefrontal (and frontal) lobes   Of the cerebral cortex, located behind the forehead, the center of human intelligence and individual personality.

psychosis   An extreme mental state, characterized by a seriously disorganized personality and reality impairment; may include auditory, visual, or tactile hallucinations or delusions.

rapid cycling   Four or more episodes (mania, hypomania, depression, mixed state) in a one-year period.

reuptake   A process of the inactivation of neurotransmitters.

serotonin   A neurotransmitter (biochemical substance) released by nerve endings in the brain that is related to mood and anxiety states.

SSRI (selective serotonin reuptake inhibitors)   Antidepressant medication that blocks the reabsorption of serotonin.

tricyclic antidepressants   The first discovered antidepressants; still very effective, but cause more side effects and toxicity than SSRIs.

UBOs (unidentified bright objects)   Suspected (but unconfirmed) small vessel damage viewed light areas on MRI brain scans.

unipolar disorder   A mood disorder; recurrent bouts of depression without cyclic episodes of mania.

Bibliography

Albom, Mitch. *Tuesdays with Morrie*. New York: Doubleday, 1997.

Bacon, Sir Francis. *Gateway to the Great Books*. Chicago: Britannica, 1963.

Beck, A., A. Rush, B. Shaw, and G. Emery. *Cognitive Therapy of Depression*. New York: Guilford Press, 1979.

Beitman, Bernard D. *Structure of Individual Psychotherapy*. New York: Guilford Press, 1987.

Bowring, M., and M. Kovacs. "Difficulties in Diagnosing Manic Disorders in Children and Adolescents." *Journal of the American Academy of Child and Adolescent Psychiatry* 31 (1992): 611–614.

Bratman, Steven, M.D. *The Alternative Medicine Ratings Guide*. Roseville, CA: Prima Publishing, 1998.

_____. *Beat Depression with St. John's Wort*. Roseville, CA: Prima Publishing, 1997.

Burlingame, Michael. *The Inner World of Abraham Lincoln*. Champagne, IL: University of Illinois Press, 1994.

Burns, D. *Feeling Good: The New Mood Therapy*. New York: Avon Books, 1992.

_____. *Ten Days to Self-Esteem*. New York: William Morrow, 1993.

Carlson, Karen J., M.D., Stephanie A. Eisenstat, M.D., and Terra Ziporyn, Ph.D. *The Harvard Guide to Women's Health*. Cambridge, MA: Harvard University Press, 1996.

Carlson, Richard, Ph.D. *Don't Sweat the Small Stuff*. New York: Hyperion, 1997.

Chandler, James, M.D., FRCPC. Web site: www.drsoft.com/chandler/pamphlet/bipolar//bipolarpamphlet.htm

Clark, David M. and Christopher G. Fairburn. *Science and Practice of Cognitive Behavioral Therapy*. New York: Oxford University Press, 1997.

Copeland, Mary Ellen, M.S. *Living Without Depression and Manic Depression*. Oakland, CA: New Harbinger, 1994.

Costello, E. "Child Psychiatric Disorders and Their Correlates: A Primary Care Pediatric Sample." *Journal of the American Academy of Child and Adolescent Psychiatry*, 28 (1989): 851–855.

Cronkite, Kathy. *On the Edge of Darkness*. New York: Delta, 1995.

Csikszentmihalyi, Mihaly. *Flow: The Psychology of Optimal Experience*. New York: HarperPerennial, 1990.

"Depression Confession." *Nation*, (June 28, 1999): 10.

Dobson, K. *The Handbook of Cognitive Therapies*. New York: Guilford Press, 1988.

Duke, Patty, and Gloria Hochman, *Brilliant Madness: Living with Manic-Depressive Illness*. New York: Bantam Books, 1992.

Esters, I., P. Cooker, and R. Ittenbach. "Effects on a Unit of Instruction in Mental Health on Rural Adolescents' Conceptions of Mental Illness and Attitudes about Seeking Help." *Adolescence* 33:130 (Summer 1998): 469–476.

Ettlinger, R.W., P. Flordh, "Attempted Suicide: Experience of 500 Cases at a General Hospital." *ACTA Psychiatr Neurol Scand*, 1955; 103 (Suppl): 1–45

Fawcett, Jan, and W.A. Scheftner, L. Fogg, D.C. Clark, M.A. Young, D. Hedeker, and R. Gibbons. "Time-Related Predictors of Suicide in Major Affective Disorder." *The American Journal of Psychiatry*, 147 (1990): 1189–1194.

Feniger, Mani. *Journey from Anxiety to Freedom*. Rocklin, CA: Prima Publishing, 1997.

Foley, Denise, and Eileen Nechas. *Women's Encyclopedia of Health and Emotional Healing*. New York: Bantam Books, 1995.

Ford, Gillian. *Listening to Your Hormones*., Rocklin, CA: Prima Publishing, 1995.

Frank, Otto. *Anne Frank: The Diary of A Young Girl*. New York: Doubleday, 1995.

Frankl, Viktor E. *Man's Search for Meaning*. New York: Pocket Books, 1963.

_____. *Man's Search for Ultimate Meaning*. Hagerstown, MD: Insight Books, 1997.

_____. *Viktor Frankl Recollections: An Autobiography*. Hagerstown, MD: Insight Books, 1995.

Freud, Sigmund. *The Interpretation of Dreams*. New York: Avon Books, 1965.

Geller, B., and J. Luby. "Child and Adolescent Bipolar Disorder: A Review of the Past 10 Years." *Journal of the American Academy of Child and Adolescent Psychiatry* 36 (1997): 1168–1176.

Gies, Miep. *Anne Frank Remembered*. New York: Simon & Schuster, 1987.

Gittelman, R., et al. "Hyperactive Boys Almost Grown Up." *Archives of General Psychiatry* 42 (1985): 937–947.

Goldfried, M., and G. Davison. *Clinical Behavior Therapy*., New York: Holt, Rinehart and Winston, 1976.

Goleman, Daniel. *Emotional Intelligence*. New York: Bantam Books, 1995.

Goodwin, Frederick K., M.D., and Tracey L. Irvin, M.D "General Guidelines and Intricacies in the Treatment of Bipolar Disorder;" and Rosenbaum, Jerrold F., M.D., and Steffany Fredman. "Medication Controversies in the Treatment of Bipolar Disorder." From the 1999 American Psychiatric Association Annual Meeting. Web site: ww.medscape.com.

Goodwin, Frederick K., M.D., and Kay Redfield Jamison, Ph.D. *Manic-Depressive Illness*. New York: Oxford University Press, 1990.

Gore, Tipper, and Rosalynn Carter. "On America's Mental Health Crisis, ." *Psychology Today* (September/October 1999).

Gray, John, Ph.D. *Men Are from Mars, Women Are from Venus*. New York: HarperCollins, 1992.

Grigoroiu-Serbanescu, M. and P.J. Wickramaratne, S.E. Hodge, S. Milea and R. Milhailescu. "Genetic anticipation and imprinting in bipolar 1 illness." *British Journal of Psychiatry*, 170:162–166 (February 1997).

Hall, Richard C.W., M.D., Dennis E. Platt, M.D., and Ryan C.W. Hall. "Suicide Risk Assessment: A Review of Risk Factors for Suicide in 100 Patients Who Made Severe Suicide Attempts." *Psychosomatics* 40 (February 1999): 18–27.

Hazell, P.L. et al."Confirmation that the Child Behavior Checklist Clinical Scales Discriminate Juvenile Mania from Attention Deficit Hyperactivity Disorder." *Journal of Pediatric Child Health*, 35:2 (1999): 199–203.

Hill, Napoleon, and W. Clement Stone. *Success Through a Positive Mental Attitude*. Chicago, IL: Prentice-Hall, 1960.

Hite, Shere. *Women & Love*. New York: St. Martin's Press, 1987.

Jamison, Kay Redfield. *Night Falls Fast*. New York: Alfred A. Knopf, 1999.

———. *Touched with Fire*. New York: Free Press, 1994.

_____. *An Unquiet Mind*. New York: Vintage Books, 1996.

Jong, Erica. *Fear of Fifty*. New York: HarperPaperbacks, 1995.

Jung, C.G. *The Undiscovered Self*. New York: Little, Brown and Company, 1957.

Kahn, Ada P., Ph.D. *Stress A-Z: A Sourcebook for Facing Everyday Challenges*. New York: Facts On File,1998.

Kahn, Ada, and Linda Hughey Holt, M.D. *Midlife Health: A Woman's Practical Guide to Feeling Good*. New York: Avon Books, 1989.

Kahn, Ada, Ph.D., and Sheila Kimmel, M.A. *Empower Yourself: Every Woman's Guide to Self-Esteem*. New York: Avon Books, 1997.

Kierkegaard, Soren. *Philosophers of the Spirit*. London: Hodder and Stoughton, 1997.

Kovacs, M., and M. Pollock. "Bipolar Disorder and Co-morbid Conduct Disorder in Childhood and Adolescence." *Journal of the American Academy of Child and Adolescent Psychiatry*, 34 (1995):; 715–723.

Kramer, Peter D. *Listening to Prozac*. New York: Penguin Books, 1994.

Krishnamurti, J. *Freedom from the Known*, New York: HarperCollins, 1969.

Kushner, Rabbi Harold S. *How Good Do We Have to Be?* New York: Little, Brown and Company, 1996.

_____. *When Bad Things Happen to Good People*. New York: Avon Books, 1983.

Lazarus, R.S., and S. Folkman. *Stress: Appraisal and Coping*. New York: Springer, 1984.

Levi, Primo. *Survival in Auschwitz*. New York: Collier Books, 1961.

Lewis, Michael. *Shame: The Exposed Self*. New York: The Free Press, 1995.

Maclaine, Shirley. *Dance While You Can*. New York: Bantam Books, 1991.

_____. *Dancing in the Light*. New York: Bantam Books, 1985.

_____. *Going Within*. New York: Bantam Books, 1989.

_____. *Out on a Limb*. New York: Bantam Books, 1983.

Masters, William H., M.D., Virginia E. Johnson, and Robert C. Kolodny, M.D. *Heterosexuality*. New York: HarperPerennial, 1992.

May, Rollo. *Existence*. New York: Basic Books, 1958.

McClellan, J., and J. Werry "Practice Parameters for the Assessment and Treatment of Children and Adolescents with Bipolar Illness." *Journal of the American Academy of Child and Adolescent Psychiatry* 36 (1997): 138–157.

Müller, Melissa. *Anne Frank: The Biography*. New York: Metropolitan Books, 1998.

Muskianth, Dr. Susan. *Depression Matters*. Johannesburg, South Africa: Delta Books, 1997.

_____. *Stress Matters*. Johannesburg: William Waterman Publications, 1996.

National Depressive and Manic-Depressive Association, "Consensus Statement on the Undertreatment of Depression." *Journal of the American Medical Association* 277:4 (January 22/29, 1997).

Opler, Lewis A., M.D., Ph.D., and Carol Bialkowski. *Prozac and Other Psychiatric Drugs*. New York: Pocket Books, 1996.

Papolos, Demitri, M.D., and Janice Papolos. *The Bipolar Child*. New York: Broadway Books, 1999.

_____. *Overcoming Depression*. New York: HarperPerennial, 1997.

Pinsky, Drew, M.D. *Restoring Intimacy: The Patient's Guide to Maintaining Relationships During Depression*. Chicago, IL: The National Depressive and Manic-Depressive Association, 1999.

Ratushinskaya, Irina. *No, I'm Not Afraid*. Newcastle upon Tyne, England: Bloodaxe Books, 1986.

Robins, Eli, G.E. Murphy, R.H. Wilkinson, et al. "Some Clinical Considerations in the Prevention of Suicide Based on a Study of 134 Successful Suicides." *American Journal of Public Health* 49 (1959): 888–899.

Rosenfeld, Nancy. *Just as Much a Woman*. Rocklin, CA: Prima Publishing, 1999.

_____. *Unfinished Journey: From Tyranny to Freedom*. Lanham, MD: University Press of America, 1993.

Rothenberg, Robert E., M.D., F.A.C.S. *The New American Medical Dictionary and Health Manual*. New York: Signet Reference, 1992.

Roy, A., G. Rylander, M. Sarchiapone, "Genetics of Suicide: Family Studies and Molecular Genetics." *Annals of New York Academy of Sciences*, December 1997; 29; 836:135–57.

Sarnii, C. *The Development of Emotional Competence*. New York: The Guilford Press, 1999.

Seligman, Martin E.P. *Learned Optimism*. New York: Pocket Books, 1998.

Sheehy, Gail. *Passages*. New York: Bantam Books, 1976.

_____. *Pathfinders*. New York: Bantam Books, 1982.

_____. *The Silent Passage: Menopause*. New York: Pocket Books, 1982.

Simopoulos, Artemis P., M.D., and Jo Robinson. *The Omega Plan*. New York: HarperCollins, 1998.

Skog, Susan. *Embracing Our Essence: Spiritual Conversations with Prominent Women*. Deerfield Beach, FL: Health Communications, Inc., 1995.

Sontag, Susan. *Illness as Metaphor and Aids and Its Metaphors*. New York: Doubleday, 1990.

Steel, Danielle. *His Bright Light*. New York: Delacorte Press, 1998.

Strober, M., et al. "A Family Study of Bipolar I Disorder in Adolescence: Early Onset of Symptoms Linked to Increased Familial Loading and Lithium Resistance." *Journal of Affective Disorders* 15 (1988): 255–268.

_____. "Recovery and Relapse in Adolescents with Bipolar Illness: A Five-Year Naturalistic Study." *Journal of the American Academy of Child and Adolescent Psychiatry* 34 (1995): 724–731.

Tarnopolsky, Yuri. *Memoirs of 1984*. Lanham, MD: University Press of America, 1993.

Taylor, Shelley E. *Positive Illusions*. New York: Basic Books, 1989.

Tejedor, M.C., A. Diaz, J.J. Castillon, J.M. Pericay. "Attempted Suicide: Repetition and Survival—Findings of a Follow-up Study." *ACTA Psychiatr Scand;* September 1999; 100; 3:205–211.

Torrey, E. Fuller, M.D., Ann E. Bowler, M.S., Edward H. Taylor, Ph.D., and Irving I. Gottesman, Ph.D. *Schizophrenia and Manic-Depressive Disorder*. New York: Basic Books, 1994.

"The Uncounted Enemy: A Vietnam Deception." CBS News Reports, 1982 documentary with Mike Wallace. Web site: www.s-t.com/daily/01-98/01-05-98/c01ae100.htm.

Weissmann, Arlene Nancy. "The Dysfunctional Attitudes Scale: A Validation Study." *Dissertation Abstracts International* (1979): 1389–1390.

Wachtler, Sol. *After the Madness: A Judge's Own Prison Memoir*. New York: Random House, 1992.

"What It Would Really Take." *Time* (June 17, 1999): 54–55.

Wiesel, Elie. *Dawn*. New York: Avon Books, 1960.

———. *Les Juifs du Silence*. Paris. Editions du Seuil, 1966.

Wolpert, Dr. Edward Alan., *Manic Depressive Illness: History of a Syndrome*. New York: International Universities Press, 1977.

Index

About the Authors

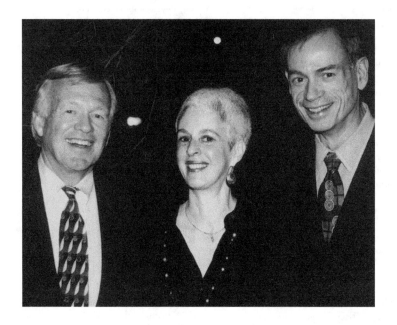

Jan Fawcett, M.D., a noted practitioner and clinical investigator, is the Stanley G. Harris Professor and chairman of psychiatry at Rush-Presbyterian-St. Luke's Medical Center, Chicago, and Grainger Director of the Rush Institute for Mental Well-Being. A graduate of Yale University Medical School, Dr. Fawcett is also the recipient of the 1999 Menninger Award for distinguished contributions to the field of mental health, and the 2000 Lifetime Research Award from the American Foundation for Suicide Prevention.

Among his many achievements, Fawcett has been the principal or co-investigator on more than 40 individual mental health research projects, including four funded grants. In 1978 he was the principle investigator of the National Institute of Mental Health's collaborative depression study. It was the beginning of a 20-year follow-up of patients diagnosed with depression and manic-depression. In 1986, he helped found the National Depressive and Manic-Depressive Association (National DMDA), and established the Dr. Jan Fawcett Humanitarian Award in 1987. The first recipient of this award was Frederick K. Goodwin.

Jan Fawcett, who is the author of four other books and one in-progress (*Manic-Depressive Illness*, 2nd Edition, Oxford University Press, 2002), is also editor of *Psychiatric Annals.*

Bernard Golden, Ph.D., a professor at the Illinois School of Professional Psychology in Chicago, has been a practicing psychologist for more than 25 years. He studied at the National Psychological Association for Psychoanalysis in New York and has worked extensively with children, adolescents, and adults in inpatient and outpatient settings. While Dr. Golden focuses on anger management, he has presented workshops on mental health issues to a wide variety of audiences. He is the author of *Healthy Anger: How to Help Children and Teens Manage Their Anger,* Oxford University Press, 2003.

Nancy Rosenfeld is the author of two other books: *Unfinished Journey: From Tyranny to Freedom,* which details her fight to free a Soviet political prisoner; and *Just As Much a Woman: Your Personal Guide to Hysterectomy and Beyond,* Prima Publishing, 1999.

After suffering a nervous breakdown in 1988, Nancy was later diagnosed with bipolar disorder. She has spent the last 10 years studying this illness to more fully understand and resolve her own issues. Nancy and her husband, Martin, reside in a Chicago suburb and have two grown sons and a grandson.